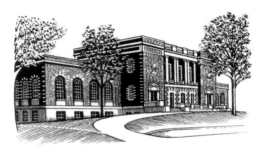
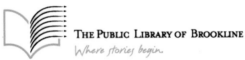

KIDS, SPORTS, AND CONCUSSION

Recent Titles in
The Praeger Series on Contemporary Health and Living

KIDS, SPORTS, AND CONCUSSION

A Guide for Coaches and Parents

SECOND EDITION

WILLIAM PAUL MEEHAN III, MD

FOREWORD BY LYLE J. MICHELI, MD

The Praeger Series on Contemporary Health and Living
Julie K. Silver, MD, Series Editor

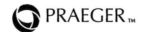

An Imprint of ABC-CLIO, LLC
Santa Barbara, California • Denver, Colorado

617.1
Meehan
2018

Copyright © 2018 by William Paul Meehan III, MD

Library of Congress Cataloging-in-Publication Data

Names: Meehan, William P., III (William Paul), author.
Title: Kids, sports, and concussion : a guide for coaches and parents /
    William Paul Meehan III, MD; foreword by Lyle J. Micheli, MD.
Description: Second edition. | Santa Barbara, California : Praeger, an imprint
    of ABC-CLIO, LLC, [2018] | Series: The Praeger series on contemporary
    health and living | Includes bibliographical references and index.
Identifiers: LCCN 2017047051 (print) | LCCN 2017047322 (ebook) |
    ISBN 9781440858031 (ebook) | ISBN 9781440858024 (print : alk. paper)
Subjects: LCSH: Sports injuries in children. | Brain—Concussion. | Child athletes—
    Wounds and injuries. | Teenage athletes—Wounds and injuries.
Classification: LCC RC1218.C45 (ebook) | LCC RC1218.C45 M44 2018 (print) |
    DDC 617.1/027083—dc23
LC record available at https://lccn.loc.gov/2017047051

ISBN: 978-1-4408-5802-4 (print)
        978-1-4408-5803-1 (ebook)

22 21 20 19 18   1 2 3 4 5

This book is also available as an eBook.

Praeger
An Imprint of ABC-CLIO, LLC

ABC-CLIO, LLC
130 Cremona Drive, P.O. Box 1911
Santa Barbara, California 93116-1911
www.abc-clio.com

This book is printed on acid-free paper ∞

Manufactured in the United States of America

For Marie, Billy, Fionnuala, and Connor

CONTENTS

FOREWORD

I am very pleased to introduce Dr. Bill Meehan's parents' and coaches' guide to sports-related concussions.

Such a book is long overdue. A true health crisis is emerging as we in the sports medicine field come to understand that far too many concussions are occurring on the sports field. What is even more disturbing is that this very dangerous injury is often not reported or is underreported. The short- and long-term implications of concussion injuries are not fully appreciated, and as a result, they are often managed in an inadequate fashion.

Dr. Meehan's book is the first book for parents on this subject. In this excellent resource, you will find information that clarifies the extent of the concussion problem, signs you can use to recognize concussions in your own child, and proper guidelines for management, monitoring, and safe return to play for the young athlete.

Although sports medicine is a relatively young discipline, there is a growing awareness of how important it is that injuries sustained by athletes receive focused assessment and management. Injuries to young athletes are of particular concern. In addition to how we diagnose and treat these injuries, there is a particular emphasis now on injury *prevention*.

Nowhere is this more important than in sports injuries to the brain. Unlike other anatomical areas such as our bones, muscles, ligaments, and tendons, our brain tissue has relatively limited ability to heal and repair itself. If not recognized and treated early on, repeated injuries to the brain can result in lasting and permanent damage. And of course, above and beyond all other tissue in our body, the brain plays a fundamental role in our ability to function as human beings.

All this makes it imperative that we focus on early recognition and diagnosis of concussion injuries, especially in our children, who depend on us for their safety. Furthermore, everyone in the sports environment—parents, coaches, team officials, and athletes—must combine their efforts to find and implement the most effective means of *preventing* injuries to the young athlete's brain.

Dr. Meehan's book will explain to parents what your role is and will help you appreciate the wide-ranging impact of such an injury on your children's lives. This extends from their ability to interact with their peers to completing homework assignments, all the way to their overall mood and behavior.

The great challenge for the next generation of sports medicine experts will be to develop systematic methods to prevent concussion in sports. This may include modified or new sports rules, coach, and official education, and even new training techniques and protective equipment.

I believe every parent will find this new book a fascinating and comprehensive look at this important subject. I give it my highest recommendation and consider it a must-read in the growing lexicon of sports medicine books for a public interested in this field.

Lyle J. Micheli, MD
Director, Division of Sports Medicine, Boston Children's Hospital
O'Donnell Family Professor of Orthopedic Sports Medicine
Clinical Professor of Orthopedic Surgery, Harvard Medical School
Past Secretary General, International Federation of Sports Medicine
Past President, American College of Sports Medicine

ACKNOWLEDGMENTS

There are countless people I need to thank for contributing, both directly and indirectly, to this second edition of *Kids, Sports, and Concussion: A Guide for Coaches and Parents*. First and foremost, I thank the athletes, patients, and health care providers at the Micheli Center for Sports Injury Prevention and the Division of Sports Medicine of Boston Children's Hospital, from whom I learn every day. I have been honored to care for thousands of athletes during my career. I am grateful to each and every one, particularly those who were kind enough to describe their experiences and offer their insights to those who read this book: Amanda Giambanco, Laura Schissler, Alyssa Paul, and Charlie Cook. I am particularly grateful to Maureen Cook, MD, who has offered a heartfelt and insightful look into the experiences of a parent determining whether or not to allow her son to participate in collision sports after sustaining a number of concussions.

Since founding the Sports Concussion Clinic, it has expanded dramatically and currently offers clinic appointments six days a week in five Boston Children's Hospital locations. I am grateful to all of the physicians who contribute to the clinic including Pierre d'Hemecourt, Andrea Stracciolini, Cynthia Stein, Mike Beasley, Ellen Geminiani, Bridget Quinn, Kate Ackerman, Joanna Fraser, Leslie Milne, Sarah Jackson, and especially Michael J. O'Brien, MD, who took over as director in 2013. I remain grateful to Lyle J. Micheli, MD, Chief of the Division of Sports Medicine, who allows us to continue both our clinical care and research efforts under his guidance. In addition, we have many collaborators in multiple departments who help us care for patients, including Mark Proctor, Alex Taylor, Karameh Kuemmerle, Jacob Brodsky, Bob Wolff, Aparna Raghuram, Ankoor Shah, Alyssa Lebel, Anna Minster, Celiane Rey-Casserly, Michel Fayad, David Fogelman, Ellen Grant, Regina Laine, Donna Nimec, Rebecca Stevens, Robert Tasker, Danielle Thurston, Sharon Chirban, Laura Moretti, Emily Pluhar, Elspeth Hart, Sara Cline, Jackie Murphy, Steph Burgess, Michele Flannery, Casey Gavin, Meghan Keating, Betsy Kramer, Mariah Mullen, Stacey Murphy, Emily Hanson, Shannon Savage, Lizanne Barone, and

Alysse Corolla. We have much needed administrative support from Maureen Piccolo, Gabi Scippa, Alyssa Aguiar, Stacey Gigante, Christine Gonzalez, Adrienne Frazier, Jill Muise, among many others.

In addition, I am privileged to work with some of the greatest sports medicine team clinicians caring for athletes in the Boston area, including Gian Corrado, Frank Wang, Amy Costa, Doug Comeau, Peter Doyle, Pete Viteritti, Carl Gustafson, Brant Berkstresser, Steve Bushee, Steve Clark, Rick Burr, Sarah Gurry, Jeanine Donato, Frank Mastrangelo, Pat Cordeiro, and Liz Cilia, among many others. Special thanks goes to Steve Bushee for sharing the concussion procedures he helped write at Boston College with the readers of this text.

There are many mentors who continue to help guide my efforts. Lyle J. Micheli, MD, is a world famous surgeon specializing in sports medicine and orthopedics. He is chief of Sports Medicine at Boston Children's Hospital, professor of orthopedics at Harvard Medical School, past president of the American College of Sports Medicine, past secretary general of the International Federation of Sports Medicine, and holds many other prominent titles. Despite his stature, he has always taken time to provide me with advice, guidance, and support. I am indebted to him for taking such an active interest in my career. Sports medicine is a division of the Department of Orthopedics, which is headed by Peter Waters, MD, who continues to give me guidance and support throughout my career, meeting with me monthly, and offering me repeated opportunities to improve my leadership skills. I remain grateful for his mentorship. In addition, I have been mentored by many senior leaders in medicine and science who have helped with both clinical and investigative efforts including Jim Kasser, Rich Bachur, Gary Fleisher, Andy Taylor, and Mark Proctor.

We are assisted in clinical research by many of the clinicians mentioned earlier as well as Dai Sugimoto, David Howell, Becky Zwicker, Chris Cuna, Natalie Slick, Bridget Dahlberg, Max McKee-Proctor, Caitlin McCracken, and Anna Brilliant, who coordinate all ongoing studies through the clinic. We have countless collaborators including Peter Kriz, Andy Taylor, Can Tan, Grant Iverson, Hamish Kerr, Jim MacDonald, Jon Minor, Tina Master, Lauren Jantzie, Dody Robinson, Marsha Moses, Dawn Comstock, Mickey Collins, Anthony Kontos, RJ Elbin, Greg Myer, Tom Buckley, Christine Baugh, Aaron Baggish, Skip Pope, Josh Easter, Steve Stache, Matt Eisenberg, Michael Monuteaux, Roger Zemek, Jeffrey Colvin, Marney Naeser, Ross Zafonte, Paul Berkner, Alex Lin, Lexi Stillman, Mo Shafi, Inga Koerte, and Marty Shenton, among many others.

We are assisted in laboratory research by my teacher and mentor, pediatric intensivist, Michael J. Whalen, and my colleagues in the lab, Jianhua Qiu, Sasha Alcon, Nick Morris, Jumana Hashim, and Grace Conley. We are grateful to our many collaborators including Ping Lu, Xiao Zhou, Alex Rotenberg, Dody Robinson, and Lauren Jantzie. Our clinical research is supported by the entire staff of the Micheli Center for Sports Injury Prevention, especially Corey Dawkins, Jen Morse, Dennis Borg, Jeff Brodeur, Sara Cline, Sara Collins,

Farren Davis, Kelsey Griffith, Mickey Cassella Kulak, Brian Mittelholzer, Mike Taksir, Felix Wang, Amy Whited, and Larry Murphy.

It is hard to know, in the context of all of these acknowledgements, where to place Rebekah Mannix, MD, MPH. She is the leader of the multidisciplinary traumatic brain injury research lab and associate director of the Brain Injury Center at Boston Children's Hospital. She is my main collaborator on all clinical research, basic science research, and outreach efforts. She is my mentor, career guide, and confidant. I owe her enormous thanks.

Most importantly, I must acknowledge the constant patience and support of my wife, Marie, who has allowed me to spend countless hours studying concussive brain injury, conducting clinical and scientific research, running the Micheli Center, co-leading the Football Players Health Study at Harvard, and preparing this book. She gave me the time I needed to dedicate to this book by keeping up our home and caring for our children. She found me a speech recognition software program to assist with writing, as I am still a hunt-and-peck typist. She provides general counsel for all of my career decisions and all of my life decisions.

To each and every person noted here, I am truly grateful.

Bill Meehan, MD

INTRODUCTION

We were in the heart of the rugby scrum. A 20-year-old lock playing for Boston College was struck in the head by a forceful kick of an opponent. As the ball was released, he staggered away toward the wrong end of the field before collapsing to the ground. He rose unsteadily, only to collapse again. Finally, he rose to his feet and began sprinting, in an attempt to rejoin the play. But he was running in the wrong direction, away from ball. He fell one last time, only to be helped off of the field by his teammates.

"What's the matter with him," hollered the coach.

"He's alright," came the reply. "He just got his bell rung."

And that was how it was.

We got "shaken up" or "had our bells rung." We simply "shook it off," "toughed it out," or "walked it off." The word *concussion* was rarely used. When it was used, it was mostly for athletes who were knocked unconscious for longer than a few seconds. Many times, we returned to the game in which we were injured. Often, we returned while still experiencing headaches, ringing in the ears, and other symptoms.

So why all the concern nowadays? What was it that changed the way sport-related concussion is diagnosis and managed? Why is the media constantly reporting stories about concussion in young athletes?

Four main medical findings change the way we think about sport-related concussion:

1. Concussion results in measurable brain dysfunction, which lasts for several days, weeks, or even months in some athletes.
2. This brain dysfunction often persists, even after the athlete reports being symptom-free.
3. Athletes who sustain one concussion are at increased risk of sustaining more concussions in the future.

4. The effects of multiple concussions are cumulative.
5. There may be long-term effects, only revealed later in life, which result from sustaining multiple concussions earlier in an athlete's career.

These recent medical findings have led to a relatively rapid change in the way doctors and other clinicians think about sport-related concussions and concussive brain injury in general. This rapid change in thinking has generated a lot of attention, not only in the medical literature, but also in the popular media. When many of us were growing up, a concussion was not thought to be serious injury. Athletes often laughed and joked about it. Certainly few people believed that there were any long-term effects or brain dysfunction that could result from a concussion or even multiple concussions.

Nowadays we know that a concussion results in a true, measurable, loss of brain function that can persist, even after athletes feel that they are completely recovered. Furthermore, we know that sustaining multiple concussions over the course of one's career can lead to more permanent brain dysfunction, depression, and other problems. This sudden change in thinking has left many athletes, parents, coaches and others confused. Some still believe the concussion is a trivial injury that can be ignored or simply shaken off, while in some circles there is a tendency to overestimate the risks involved in participating in sports that carry a high risk of concussion. Such over estimations have led to calls to ban sports altogether or to ban certain collision sports such as American football and ice hockey. This book will help clarify the medical and scientific data that have resulted in this change of thinking. In doing so, this book will answer the following questions:

- What is a concussion?
- How common is concussion?
- Can an athlete prevent a concussion?
- What is the best way to assess a concussion?
- What can be done to treat a concussion?
- When is it safe to return to playing after a concussion?
- What are the risks of suffering multiple concussions?
- Are there ways of preventing or decreasing the potential effects of multiple concussions?
- Is ethical to allow children to participate in sports that carry a high risk of concussion?

In addition, readers of this book will learn how they can respond to a concussed athlete, as well as what they should expect from medical personnel tending to a concussed athlete. For those readers interested in starting a comprehensive concussion management program in their area, this book contains some recommendations on how to proceed. In addition, the book contains the stories of several athletes describing, in their own words, their experiences with concussions. This new, second edition of this book, also contains a very insightful story by a mother and physician who was forced to decide whether she should allow her son to return to American football after he had sustained multiple concussions.

At the end of each chapter is a list of suggested readings for those readers who may wish to learn more about the topics covered within the chapter. Many of these readings are medical or scientific articles, often those referred to in the chapter. While these articles may use some medical and scientific jargon, I believe the overall principles can be appreciated, even without scientific or medical training.

Lastly, chapter 18 contains the definitions of terms commonly used in sports medicine and brief descriptions of common occupations in the field of sports medicine. This chapter can serve as a reference for the reader unfamiliar with the field.

1

WHAT IS A CONCUSSION?

On October 30, 1974, the world heavyweight champion, George Foreman, fought Muhammad Ali in a bout that will forever be remembered as "the rumble in the jungle." Many readers my age or older will remember watching this fight on television or seeing the countless replays of it over the last 43 years. The fight was memorable for many reasons. It was only the second time in heavyweight history a former champion reclaimed the title. It introduced Don King to the world as a professional boxing promoter. The fight took place in Zaire, in central Africa, a country now known as the Democratic Republic of Congo. It ended with controversy as some argue that Foreman was counted out despite being on his feet by the count of nine. But perhaps the "rumble in the jungle" is most remembered for the strategy Ali used during the fight, which has come to be known as "rope a dope."

Early in the fight, Ali began lying against the ropes, allowing George Foreman to deliver multiple blows. He mounted few attacks against the reigning champion. He dodged many of Foreman's thrusts. He blocked many aside. He allowed several of the less powerful blows to land on relatively harmless areas of the body. He tangled Foreman up, and wrestled with him. He taunted Foreman, challenging him to throw harder, more vicious blows. Foreman, who was recognized as the more powerful fighter, seemed only too happy to oblige. As the fight went on, however, the amount of energy Foreman spent trying to land these powerful blows, and trying to disentangle himself from Ali, took its toll. He was visibly tired at the start of the eighth round.

In fact, the beginning, if not most, of the eighth round seemed little different from the prior rounds. Ali allowed Foreman to punch away, only occasionally offering a quick straight jab to Foreman's face. But as the round neared its end, with only 18 seconds remaining, Ali unleashed a flurry of blows. In the final combination, Ali stood Foreman nearly upright with a left hook to the face. Foreman's left hand dropped to his side, exposing his chin to a punishing right cross that Ali landed squarely on Foreman's jaw. With only 12 seconds remaining in the round, Foreman, staggered, fell, and was counted out, ending the fight.

George Foreman had been concussed.

But why? What is it that happened to George Foreman's brain at the time of that right cross that rendered him stunned, off-balance, incapable of continuing the fight? What was it about that right cross that resulted in Foreman's brain malfunctioning? If the brain is located in the top of the head, above the eyes, why would a punch to the jaw injure the brain at all? This chapter will provide answers to these questions.

A concussion is a type of traumatic brain injury. When athletes sustain concussions, their brains stop functioning properly as a result of trauma. Perhaps the simplest way to think of a sport-related concussion is: a temporary dysfunction of the brain caused by trauma.

Despite popular belief, a concussion is not a bruise on the brain. There is no detectable bruising, bleeding, or swelling of the brain by conventional, modern-day imaging of the brain. It is not cut, scratched, or abraded. The brain, however, cannot function properly when it is concussed. Memory, concentration, reaction time, the ability to learn new information, and the ability to solve problems are all temporarily disrupted when an athlete sustains a concussion.

Since one of the main functions of the brain is to maintain consciousness, any athlete who loses consciousness after head trauma has sustained a concussion. Most concussions in sports, however, do not involve a loss of consciousness. In fact, less than 10% of all sport-related concussions involve a loss of consciousness.

A blow dealt to the shoulder will bruise the shoulder. Most people are familiar with this type of injury. Therefore, many people believe that a concussion is a bruise on the brain sustained by a blow to the head. Medical science, however, has shown that this is not true. Remember, the brain is protected by the thick, hard bone of the skull. In order to bruise the brain, the skull would have to break or bend inward and strike the brain. While this can happen, the forces involved in sports are often too low to cause this type of skull deformity. Furthermore, in the sports that carry the greatest risk for sustaining concussions, the brain is often protected by a hard helmet in addition to the skull. In fact, many concussions are caused by a blow to the facemask, chin, or other part of the body, as opposed to the head. Readers who are familiar with boxing or mixed martial arts will be well aware of this. Concussions are fairly common in these sports. For a physician who studies concussive brain injury, a lot can be learned from observing these combat sports.

At the time of writing the first edition of this book, I was having trouble sleeping. I used to get out of bed, go into the living room, and watch some television. One night, I came across a show featuring the ultimate fighting championship's (UFCs) greatest knockouts. I started watching volume 3. I was on volume 6 by the time I returned to bed. There were approximately five or six knockouts per episode. So I was able to observe a good number of knockouts in a relatively short period of time. I noticed that most of these knockouts resulted from a blow to the chin. Remember that the brain is in the top of the skull, mostly above the eyes. A blow to the chin results in no impact on the brain whatsoever. It does, however, result in a significant movement or "spinning" of the brain at the time of impact. As we shall soon see, it is this rapid movement of the brain that results in a concussion.

So what is it that causes a concussion?

A concussion is caused by an acceleration of the brain. After the head, face, or other part of the body is struck, the brain is sent spinning in the opposite direction. For example, if a basketball player is struck on the left side of the face by the elbow of an opponent, his or her head will accelerate to the right. This rapid movement, or acceleration, of the brain causes it to malfunction. In particular, rotational acceleration or spinning of the brain results in a concussion.

There are two main ways to accelerate something. You can push it in a straight line, such that it accelerates in a straight line, away from your pushing hand. This type of acceleration is known as linear acceleration. Imagine a car at a stoplight along a straight road. When the light turns green, the driver steps on the gas. The car starts from a complete stop and accelerates, in a straight line, until the driver reaches a cruising speed at 25–30 miles per hour. This is a form of linear acceleration.

Alternatively, you can accelerate something by spinning it. "Spinning" is a more common term for rotational acceleration. When a child takes a toy top or dreidel, places it on a table, and spins it, the child is, in scientific terms, applying a rotational acceleration to the top. It is this rotational type of acceleration, when sustained by the human brain, that results in concussion. This has been demonstrated in scientific experiments carried out over the last century.

In some sense, it has been known for over 100 years that in order to sustain a concussion, the head has to be free to move. As often happens, this was first realized in the world outside of medicine. This knowledge was commonly used in slaughter houses. In order to prepare various meats for market, the animals must first be killed. This takes place in slaughter houses. It was thought, even 100 years ago, to be inhumane to simply walk up to the animal and kill it. Therefore, men who worked in slaughter houses used to try to stun the animal or knock it unconscious prior to killing it and butchering it in preparation for the market. One common method used to stun the animal was to deliver a concussion by striking it on the head with a bolt. Certainly, if the animal's head was held in place, preventing it from moving, it would be quite easy to strike it with the bolt. By holding the head still, the butcher could maintain the head in precisely the location where the bolt would be striking from above. Men working in slaughter houses observed, however, that if the animal's head was held in place, and not free to move after the impact, the animal would not be stunned. It would not be concussed. It would not lose consciousness. But, if the animal was held in place by the shoulders and torso, so that the head was free to move after it was struck by the bolt, the animal would often be concussed; it would be dazed, off-balance, and even frankly knocked unconscious. Once the animal was stunned from its concussion, the business of the day could proceed.

In the 1940s, this realization came to the medical community. Two researchers, named Denny-Brown and Russell, were studying concussion in animals. In order to concuss the animals, they would strike them in the head with a weight attached to a pendulum. The weight would be dropped from various heights. It would swing down and strike the animal in the head. From their experiments, we have learned that if the head is held in place, and not allowed to move after it is struck, there are cuts or lacerations of the scalp, sometimes broken skull bones, and sometimes bleeding in the brain. The brain, however, seems to function properly. The animal is upset and angry, but does not appear stunned, dazed, disoriented, and is seldom knocked unconscious. If, however, the head is free to move after it has been struck, the brain stops functioning properly. The animals often lose consciousness or "get knocked out." Even when they do not get knocked unconscious, they are clearly off-balance and dazed. This led physicians and scientists to believe that it was not the blow itself that causes a concussion, but rather, the rapid movement of the brain after the blow, the acceleration of the brain.

Over time, other medical and scientific research confirmed these findings: the head must accelerate after impact in order for a concussion to occur. This observation led doctors and scientists to conclude that it is the acceleration of the brain that leads to a concussion as opposed to the impact itself. But whether it was linear acceleration or rotational acceleration that led to the injury remained unknown.

Around that same time, some other observations were made. The brain consists mostly of water. Perhaps as a result, many of the physical properties of the brain are similar to those of water. For a moment, think about what would happen to a bowl of water with feathers floating on top if you were to slide it along a slippery surface, such as a piece of ice. By sliding it, you would be, in scientific terms, applying a linear acceleration to it. Once the bowl stopped sliding, the water would continue to accelerate toward the front of the bowl, climbing up its frontward surface. The water would then flow down the front surface across the bowl and up the back side of the bowl. This would ultimately lead to waves throughout the water. The feathers would bob up and down on top of the waves. But the relative positions of the feathers to one another would remain the same. Each feather would remain in more or less in the same place within the bowl, bobbing up and down on top of the waves until the waves came to a stop. If, however, you were to spin the bowl instead of sliding it in a straight line, feathers would be thrown around the bowl ending up in various locations. By spinning it, you would be, in scientific terms, applying a rotational acceleration to it.

A similar thought experiment to this was carried out by a physicist named Holburn in the 1940s. In order to follow up on this thought experiment, Holburn made a gelatin model of the brain, a fake brain made of a substance similar to Jello. He put this gelatin brain inside a wax model of a skull. He then spun the skull and brain, or, in scientific terms, he applied a rotational acceleration to the skull and brain. He then cracked open the wax skull and removed the fake brain. He saw extensive damage to it. He described the location of the damage sustained by his gelatin brain and published his findings in a medical journal, the *Lancet.* This led him as well as other scientists and physicians to believe that "spinning" a brain caused more of a problem than simply accelerating it in a straight line. However, the debate over whether rotational acceleration of the brain was more harmful than linear acceleration continued for some time.

More than 30 years after Holburn's experiment, the debate was taken up again. In order to better determine the effects of linear and rotational acceleration on the brain, two scientists, named Ommaya and Gennarelli, took the experiments one step further. They produced concussion without ever striking the brain. They separated 24 monkeys in two groups. The monkeys were each placed in a helmet, snugly affixed to the monkeys' heads. For 12 of the monkeys, they used a mechanical device, to move the helmet rapidly forward, in a straight line, one inch. All of the monkeys who underwent this linear acceleration of one inch appeared well afterward. They did not appear confused, off-balance, or dazed. They did not lose consciousness.

The remaining 12 monkeys were placed in helmets as well. But this time, the helmets were spun or rotated over an arc of one inch, using the exact same amount of force. This rapid rotational acceleration resulted in all 12 monkeys being immediately knocked unconscious. Note, there was no blow to the brain; the animals were not struck in any way. Their heads were simply accelerated either in a purely linear or purely rotational direction. Thus, this experiment confirmed that it was not simply the rapid movement or acceleration of the brain that produced the concussion, but rather the spinning or "rotational acceleration," which resulted in concussive brain injury.

More recently, video analysis of concussions and studies performed on players from the National Football League revealed that most concussive injuries are caused when a player is struck on the side of the helmet or face mask. In fact, the facemask often acts as fulcrum, causing a more rapid acceleration of the brain than blows to the shell of the helmet. Such a blow, results in a rotational acceleration of the brain, or spinning of the brain, in the opposite direction of the blow.

In many ways, a blow to the facemask and a blow to the chin result in a similar action on the brain. Let us consider for a moment a boxer striking one of his opponents. If a powerful blow is landed in the middle of the head, say just above the left ear, it may cause a lateral bending of the neck. The neck may be stretched, such that the boxer's head bends down toward the right, with the right ear moving down toward the right shoulder. If, however, the boxer throwing the punch manages to land his blow on the chin, side of the face, or side of his opponent's forehead, the head of the boxer struck will spin very rapidly toward the right. Thus, the athlete struck more toward the front of the head is more likely to sustain a concussion than the athlete struck in the middle of the head. Those of you seeking confirmation for this need merely watch ultimate fighting championships greatest knockouts, YouTube videos of fights that result in a knockout, or ESPN's classic bouts in which one of the boxers is knocked out.

The facemask extends even farther from the center of the head toward the front of the athlete. Similar to boxers, if a football player is struck in the center of his helmet, say just above the left ear hole, again the head will bend down toward the opposite shoulder. Its acceleration will be restrained somewhat by the neck musculature, which will resist bending in that direction. If, however, the football player is struck on the front of his face mask, the head will spin very rapidly in the opposite direction. Therefore, blows dealt to the front of the helmet or facemask are more likely to result in a concussion than a blow dealt to the center of the helmet.

It should be pointed out that, while rotational acceleration or spinning of the brain leads to a concussion, the spinning may occur in multiple different directions. For example, imagine a boxer who is struck by an uppercut. If the uppercut lands directly on the under surface of his chin, his head will spin upward, such that his face accelerates from its starting position, facing his opponent, upward, so that ultimately he is facing the ceiling. Thus, his head accelerates or spins in an upward direction. If, however, that same boxer is struck by a right cross that lands on his left cheek, his head would spin over his right shoulder. As opposed to spinning upward, his head would be spinning toward the right. In either case, he could sustain a concussion. So long as the brain is spinning, accelerating in a rotational fashion, a concussion can occur.

In life, most blows to the head result in rotational accelerations in several directions. It is rare for an uppercut to land directly in the center of the chin, accelerating the brain perfectly upward. More often the blow is landed on the undersurface of one side of the chin or other, which accelerates the brain upward but also off to the side. Similarly, in most real-life situations, there is both a linear and a rotational acceleration present. It is the rotational component of the acceleration, however, that causes the concussion.

So, now we know that concussion is caused by a rotational acceleration or "spinning" of the brain. But what happens to the brain, when it is spun, that prevents it from working properly?

To understand that, we must understand a little bit about how the brain works. But first, it will help us to consider some common, everyday phenomena that are analogous to the workings of the brain cells. Many readers will be familiar with what happens to a rope when one end is raised and then rapidly lowered. An upside down "U" shape appears in the rope, and travels down its length, until it reaches the end. In this way, an "impulse" can be transmitted from one end of a rope to the other end (Figure 1.1).

In some sense, the cells of the brain work similarly. The brain consists of a collection of special cells called nerve cells or "neurons." These nerve cells control all of our movements, thoughts, and bodily functions such as breathing. Each nerve cell consists of a cell body and an axon. The axon is a long, narrow part of the nerve cell used to transmit messages to other parts of the

Figure 1.1
Impulse Movement along the Length of a Rope

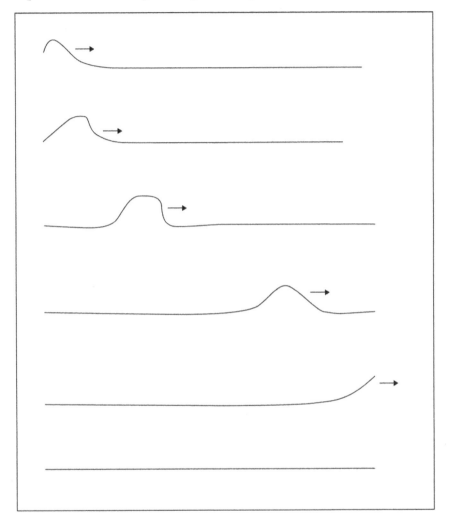

brain and other parts of the body. Nerve cells work, in part, by the movement of small molecules, called electrolytes. Most athletes will be familiar with the electrolytes sodium and potassium, which are commonly lost through sweat, and replaced by sports drinks such as Gatorade. Movement of these electrolytes along the nerve cells is essential for normal brain function.

Usually sodium and potassium are on opposite sides of the cell membrane, the outer lining of the cell (Figure 1.2). Specifically, sodium is on the outside; potassium is on the inside. In a normal functioning neuron, the cell can

Figure 1.2
A Neuron Conducting a Message

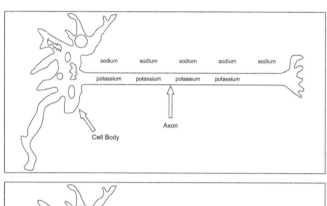

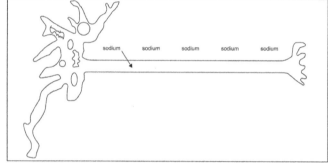

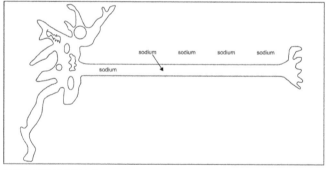

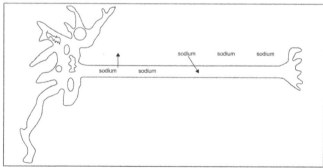

Figure 1.2 Continued

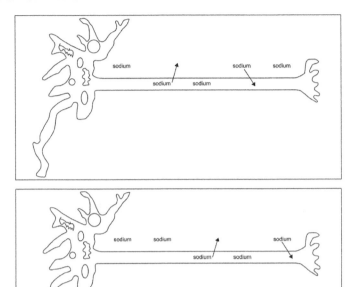

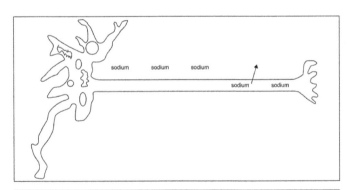

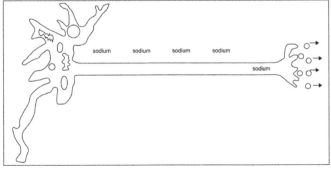

conduct messages down its axon by movement of these electrons across its membrane. When stimulated, a nerve cell will allow sodium to move into the cell from the outside (Figure 1.2). When this occurs at the start of the axon, it stimulates the adjacent area to do the same: allow sodium in. Very rapidly, the sodium is pumped back to the outside of the cell. As sodium is moving into the cell at one part of the axon, it is being returned to the outside of the cell in the previous part of the axon. This occurs all the way down the length of the axon. Thus, this "impulse" is transmitted rapidly down the length of the axon, much like the impulse started on the rope discussed earlier is transported all the way down the length of the rope. When the person holding the rope raises and lowers it rapidly, he creates an impulse that transmits down the length of the rope. As one portion of the rope rises from its resting position, the other part of the rope returns to where it was previously. Although, I am sure it seems complicated when reading about it in a paragraph, Figures 1.1 and 1.2 should go a long way in helping to understand this concept.

When this exchange of ions across the membrane, or "impulse," reaches the end of the neuron, a chemical is secreted, sending a message to the next neuron.

That is how the brain normally functions. But, when an athlete sustains a concussion, the locations of sodium and potassium are disrupted. The channels in the cell membrane that allow sodium and potassium to move across it are usually closed except when it is time to conduct a message. When a rotational acceleration of the brain is of a sufficient force to produce a concussion, these channels are opened and large amounts of sodium move into the cell, while potassium moves out of the cell. Because such large amounts move across the membrane, it takes a long time to restore them to the proper positions. The nerve cell cannot operate normally until the sodium and potassium ions are put back in their normal place, with sodium outside the cell membrane and potassium inside the cell membrane. During this time, the brain is concussed. It cannot function properly. In order to restore sodium and potassium to their normal positions along the cell membrane, the brain needs energy. Normally, energy is delivered to the brain through the bloodstream. Ironically, some experiments have shown that there is decreased blood flow to the brain after it has sustained a concussion. Thus, the brain receives less energy, at a time when it needs more energy. It is believed that this mismatch, between the need for more energy and the delivery of less energy, results in some of a patient's post-concussion symptoms.

Knowing a little bit about how the brain works is helpful. But how can you tell if an athlete has sustained concussion?

Concussion can be detected by various *signs* and *symptoms*. *Symptoms* are the feelings or problems experienced by an athlete who has sustained a concussion. Common symptoms of concussion are headaches, nausea, difficulty balancing, difficulty concentrating, and amnesia (the inability to remember things that occurred around the time of injury). Some of the most common symptoms of concussion are listed in Table 1.1.

Table 1.1
Common Symptoms of a Sport-Related Concussion

Symptoms of Concussion
• Headache
• Dizziness
• Difficulty concentrating
• Nausea or vomiting
• Difficulty balancing
• Vision changes
• Sensitivity to light
• Sensitivity to noise
• Feeling "out of it"
• Ringing in the ears
• Drowsiness
• Sadness

In addition to the symptoms experienced by the athlete, *signs* of concussion may be noticed by coaches, parents, and teammates. *Signs* are observations made by others, about an athlete who has sustained a concussion. Common signs observed in athletes who have sustained a concussion are poor balance or coordination, running the wrong play, vomiting, appearing glassy-eyed, seeming confused, or asking the same question over and over again despite being given the answer previously. Some common signs of concussion are listed in Table 1.2.

In order to help athletic trainers, doctors, and other medical personnel assess these signs and symptoms, standard lists have been developed. An athlete who has sustained an injury can rank these symptoms on what is known as a "symptom scale," or "symptom inventory." Symptom scales are often used to monitor an athlete's recovery. The Sport Concussion Assessment Tool version 5 (SCAT 5) contains a common symptom scale endorsed by the International Olympic Committee, the Fédération Internationale de Football Association (FIFA), International Rugby Board, International Ice Hockey Federation, and the Fédération Equestre Internationale. The SCAT 5 is available online at: http://bjsm.bmj.com/content/bjsports/early/2017/04/26/bjsports-2017-097506SCAT5.full.pdf.

People often wonder whether there are tests that can be performed to know for sure whether an athlete has a concussion. While there are no perfect tests for concussion, there are some that can help determine whether an athlete has sustained a concussion. Some of these tests are used to assess whether there is another reason that might explain the athlete's symptoms. These tests should

Table 1.2
Common Signs of a Sport-Related Concussion

Symptoms of Concussion
• Loss of consciousness
• Amnesia, or forgetfulness
• Walking off-balance
• Acting disoriented
• Appearing dazed
• Acting confused
• Forgetting game rules or play assignments
• Inability to recall score or opponent
• Inappropriate emotionality
• Poor physical coordination
• Slow verbal responses
• Personality changes

be normal if the athlete's symptoms are due to a concussion. Other tests are used to determine the degree to which an athlete's brain has been concussed. These tests will often be abnormal after an athlete sustains a concussion.

Many readers will be familiar with pictures of the brain or medical images such as computed tomography (CT) scans or magnetic resonance images (MRIs). CT scans and MRIs are similar to x-rays. They are types of pictures used by doctors to help determine whether a body part, such as the brain, has sustained a structural injury. These pictures can often tell whether a body part has been bruised, broken, lacerated, swollen, or sustained other traumatic injury. Unlike an x-ray, these pictures allow doctors see soft tissues, such as the brain, in addition to bone.

As there is no gross bruising, bleeding, or swelling of the brain when an athlete sustains a concussion, these pictures of the brain, CT scans and MRIs, will be normal. A doctor cannot "see" a concussion by looking at these images. When such images are obtained, these types of images will be ordered by the doctor in order to make sure there is not another injury, in addition to the concussion, that explains some of the athlete's symptoms. They are very useful in making sure the athlete does not have bleeding in the brain, swelling of the brain, or a skull fracture. Many times, however, these types of images will not be necessary.

Similarly, there is no blood test or other type of medical test that can definitively diagnose a concussion. Several possible blood tests have been studied by medical researchers. As of the time of this writing, however, none has proved effective in definitively diagnosing a concussive brain injury. Currently, at Children's Hospital Boston, there is medical research being conducted in order to identify tests from the blood, tests from the urine, tests of the cerebral spinal fluid, and other types of pictures or images that may help doctors in definitively diagnosing concussive brain injury. Until such tests have been discovered and thoroughly evaluated the context of concussion, doctors must rely, in part, on athletes reporting their symptoms to us. As many athletes do not understand concussion, or even recognize a concussion when it occurs, they often do not report their symptoms. Furthermore, many who do recognize that their symptoms are due to a concussion are so anxious to get back to play that they pretend to feel better in order to get cleared for participation. Thus, it can often be difficult to determine whether an athlete has sustained a concussion. It can be even more challenging to determine when exactly an athlete has recovered from a concussion.

Fortunately, there are some tests that can be helpful in determining whether athlete has sustained a concussion as well as when an athlete has recovered from a concussion. The neurological physical examination may reveal certain findings that are inconsistent with concussion and may cause doctors to look for other potential causes of an athlete's signs or symptoms. There are standard ways of measuring athletes' balance. Brain function can be measured. Neuropsychological or neurocognitive tests measure brain function, such as memory, the ability to concentrate, the speed with which an athlete is able to figure out problems, and reaction time, among others. Each of these tests can be used to assist clinicians in diagnosing a concussion. They will be discussed in detail in later chapters.

It is understandably frustrating for doctors, parents, coaches, and athletes that no medical test can definitively diagnose a concussion. Many of the symptoms of concussion can also be caused by other medical conditions. For example, headaches, dizziness, trouble balancing, irritability, and drowsiness can all be caused by dehydration. Headaches, nausea, sensitivity to light, and sensitivity to noise can be observed in patients with migraine headaches or athletes with a hangover, a not uncommon entity among collegiate athletes. Patients who suffer from clinical depression often feel sad, with decreased energy. Doctors must therefore understand the circumstances that resulted in the athlete's symptoms, how the symptoms have changed since they started, and other medical problems the athlete has. All of these factors will help clinicians determine whether an athlete has sustained a sport-related concussion.

Almost all assessments in medicine start with what is known as the history. The history refers to the patient's or athlete's description of how the injury occurred, how his or her symptoms started, and how the symptoms have changed since they started. After listening to patients describe their injuries and the symptoms that are bothering them, doctors often ask a series of questions to get more information. Some common questions asked by doctors to help them obtain further history are:

- When did the symptoms first start?
- Have they changed since you first noticed them?
- Are there certain things that make your symptoms worse?

- Are there certain things that make your symptoms better?
- Have you ever experienced symptoms like this before?
- Have your symptoms become worse since they first started? Have they become better since they first started?
- Are your symptoms affected by exercise?
- Are your symptoms affected by studying or other activities that demand mental concentration or focus?

By answering these questions as accurately as possible, athletes help their doctors determine whether it is likely they have sustained a concussion. Sometimes at the end of this question and answer session, it is clear that the athlete has sustained a concussion. For example, let us suppose an athlete says to his doctor:

I was playing ice hockey a week ago. I felt great at the start of the game. I was in the best shape of my life. My team was playing for the number one spot in the division. I was behind my opponent's goal when I briefly lost control of the puck. As I was looking down at the ice, trying to regain control of the puck, I was struck by one of the opposing defensemen. I didn't see the blow coming. He lifted me off my skates. The back of my head struck the boards as I fell. My head bounced off the ice. The next thing I remember I was being helped off the ice by one of my teammates and the athletic trainer. They told me I had been knocked unconscious for a few seconds. I had a killer headache and felt a little woozy. After a few minutes I started throwing up. The athletic trainer was concerned. He put a brace on my neck and had the ambulance take me to the emergency department. The doctor there ordered a CT of my brain which he told me was normal. He said I had a concussion and should stay out of hockey. And he told me to follow up here with you. Since then I've been feeling a lot better. I still get headaches almost every day, but they are not half as bad as they were first few days after I got hurt. I still have a little bit of trouble sleeping. My girlfriend says I still seem a little bit out of it from time to time. But I feel a whole lot better than I did the first few days after injury.

In this example it is clear that the athlete has sustained a sport-related concussion. He was feeling great at the start of the game, without any symptoms at all. He sustained a rapid blow to the body, followed by two blows to the head. He developed the immediate onset of headaches, nausea, confusion, and other symptoms that have gradually been improving, but have not yet completely gone away. He has had a CT of his brain which was normal, letting the doctor know that there was no bleeding in the brain, bruising of the brain, swelling of the brain, or other injuries that are causing his symptoms.

Sometimes, as in this example, it is easy to know whether an athlete sustained a concussion. At times, however, it can be more difficult. For example, suppose the athlete instead said to his doctor:

I had been sick for a few days before the game. A lot of the guys on the team felt sick. Some had vomiting. Others had diarrhea. Some had both. Still, I felt good enough to play. As the game went on, I started to get a headache. I noticed I felt a little nauseous.

At one point I skated over to the bench and told the athletic trainer I wasn't feeling well. He had me sit down and gave me some Gatorade. I threw up a couple of times and he became concerned. He thought maybe I had suffered a concussion. I don't remember taking any specific big hits to the head, but I did get banged around a few times. Anyway, my athletic trainer wanted me to come see you to get checked out. I've been feeling better over the last few days but I still don't feel 100% back to normal. I feel a little out of it, at times. I think I just caught a stomach bug.

In this situation, it is much more challenging to tell whether the athlete has sustained a sport-related concussion. Certainly, a concussion can cause an athlete to have headaches, feel nauseous, vomit, and feel "out of it." It could be that this athlete sustained sport-related concussion and that this concussion is the cause of his symptoms. But the symptoms could also be due to a stomach virus. Indeed, many of the other players on this athlete's team have recently been suffering from what seems like a stomach virus. The athlete himself felt ill, even before the game started. It could be he came down with the same illness. Further complicating the picture, he may have come down with the same viral illness that his teammates had *and* sustained a sport-related concussion. He may be suffering from both. In this case, it is much harder to tell whether the athlete has sustained a sport-related concussion. His doctor may perform further tests and assessments to help make that determination.

Once it has been determined that an athlete has sustained a sport-related concussion, the athlete, the coaches, and the parents often ask what "grade" concussion the athlete has suffered. Similarly, when I hear news reports about professional athletes who sustain concussions, the reporter often refers to the grade of the concussion. Statements such as, "the cougars will be at a distinct disadvantage this weekend as their star quarterback is out injured after having suffered a grade 2 concussion," are common. However, those of us practicing sports medicine no longer grade concussions. The terminology is mostly still used due to historical reasons.

Historically, concussions were graded. A grade 1 concussion was thought to be milder than a grade 2. Grade 3 concussions were thought to be more severe than either grade 1 or grade 2. Several factors were used to determine the grade of a concussion. Athletes who lost consciousness at the time of their concussion received a higher grade than those that did not. Athletes who were knocked unconscious for longer periods of time received higher grades than those who were unconscious for shorter amounts of time. Athletes who suffered amnesia as part of their concussions were given a higher grade than those who did not; the longer the period of time for which the athlete had a loss of memory, the higher the grade of concussion. These grades were used to determine how long an athlete should be removed from sports after sustaining a sport-related concussion. This was a very convenient system for doctors and other clinicians managing sport-related concussions. Clinicians could simply look up the grade of an athlete's concussion, ask how many concussions the athlete had sustained previously, and use standard guidelines that specified how long the athlete should remain out of play before returning to his or her sport. It turned out, however, that this approach was not the best for athletes. Some were held out of play, unnecessarily, even after full recovery. Others were put back to play too soon, prior to full recovery.

A NOTE ABOUT GRADING SYSTEMS: While grading systems have been abandoned in favor of more individualized management, they were extremely beneficial during their time. When the first grading systems were developed, few medical professionals took concussion seriously. Athletes were often sent straight back into play after sustaining a concussion, without another thought. These grading systems were instrumental in drawing much needed attention to the issue of concussive brain injury in sports. They allowed many athletes to recover from their injuries, prior to being returned to sports and risking an additional concussion.

Grading systems were abandoned in the consensus and agreement statement from the First International Conference on Concussion in Sports, which was published in 1999. Those clinicians involved in the assessment and management of sport-related concussions had noticed that athletes who were knocked unconscious for brief periods of time often recovered more quickly than those who did not lose consciousness. Therefore, it seemed inaccurate to diagnose those who did not lose consciousness with a lower grade of concussion. Furthermore, grades were used to determine the period of time that an athlete was removed from sports. It did not make sense to keep those who recovered more quickly out of sports for longer periods of time than those who recovered more slowly. For this and for several other reasons, the use of grading systems was abandoned. Nowadays, when making decisions to return an athlete back to play after he or she has recovered from a sport-related concussion, doctors consider each case individually. Rather than simply looking up a standard guideline in a book, doctors take the whole clinical picture into consideration. Factors that may help determine the amount of time an athlete is asked to remain symptom free before returning to contact include:

- The length of time over which the athlete had symptoms from the concussion
- The length of time it took for the athlete to recover his or her brain function after the concussion
- The length of time it took the athlete to recover his or her balance after the concussion
- The amount of brain dysfunction associated with the athlete's concussion
- The intensity of symptoms suffered by the athlete after the concussion
- The number of concussions the athlete has sustained over his or her lifetime
- The amount of time that elapsed in between the athlete's concussions
- The amount of force that was required to produce concussive brain injury in the athlete
- Whether the amount of force required to produce a concussion in the athlete has changed over time
- The age of the athlete
- The sport to which the athlete hopes to return

All of these factors help determine the degree of injury sustained by the athlete. They help make decisions about how much recovery time is required for an individual athlete after a sport-related concussion. They factor into decisions about when to return an athlete to contact or collision sports. They also factor into decisions about whether an athlete should ever be returned to contact or collision sports.

In summary, a concussion is a traumatic injury of the brain. It results from a rapid, rotational acceleration or spinning of the brain. It is a functional injury to the brain, meaning that the brain is not able to work properly when it is concussed. However, a concussion does not result in gross bleeding, bruising, swelling, or other structural injury to the brain. The brain cannot work properly after a concussion because the electrolytes that help the brain operate under normal circumstances have been disturbed. The severity of a concussion cannot be determined at the time of injury but rather is determined by assessing the factors that led to the injury in the first place and monitoring the length of time required for the athlete to completely recover.

Suggested Readings

Aubry, M., et al. Summary and agreement statement of the First International Conference on Concussion in Sport, Vienna, 2001. Recommendations for the improvement of safety and health of athletes who may suffer concussive injuries. *Br J Sports Med*, 2002, 36(1): 6–10.

Giza, C. C., and D. A. Hovda. The neurometabolic cascade of concussion. *J Athl Train*, 2001, 36(3): 228–235.

Holbourn, A. Mechanics of head injury. *The Lancet*, 1943, 2: 438–441.

McCrory, P., et al. Consensus statement on concussion in sport: the Fifth International Conference on Concussion in Sport held in Berlin, October 2016. *Br J Sports Med*, 2017 [Epub ahead of print].

Ommaya, A. K., and T. A. Gennarelli. Cerebral concussion and traumatic unconsciousness: Correlation of experimental and clinical observations of blunt head injuries. *Brain*, 1974, 97(4): 633–654.

Shaw, N. A. The neurophysiology of concussion. *Prog Neurobiol*, 2002, 67(4): 281–344.

2

Sport-Related Concussion: How Common It Is

On October 27, 2007, the Philadelphia Flyers were playing the Boston Bruins. The score was 0 to 0 with 3:53 remaining in the first period. The puck was sent from just over the center line to behind the Flyers net. Boston Bruin, Patrice Bergeron, and Philadelphia Flyer, Randy Jones, skated after it. Bergeron arrived there first, sending the puck to his right, around the back of the net. Jones finished his body check on Bergeron, striking him from behind. Bergeron's face was thrown up against the edge of the dasher board. Jones's momentum carried him into Bergeron, compressing the Bruin's head into the boards further. Bergeron fell on the ice. He was motionless. He was unconscious.

Patrice Bergeron was concussed.

This case drew a great deal of media attention, particularly in the Boston area. It illustrated several poorly understood points about sport-related concussion. First of all, Patrice Bergeron missed the majority of the remaining hockey season due to his concussion. For many sports fans at the time, a concussion was thought to be a minor injury that might cause an athlete to miss, at most, one week of play. Furthermore, this concussion occurred during ice hockey. American football receives a larger share of the medical and sports media attention regarding sport-related concussions. Given the large number of athletes playing football, more football players sustain sport-related concussions in any given year than do the athletes of other team sports. However, as we shall see, the proportion of ice hockey players sustaining a concussion over a given season is comparable to if not greater than that of the American football players.

This chapter will discuss many of the sports during which concussions occur. The relative frequency of concussion in each will be described. When known, various activities of the sport that increase the risk of concussion will be reviewed. Comparisons between male and female athletes playing the same sport will also be considered.

Sport-related concussion is a common injury. Exactly how common depends on the sport being played, the level of competition, the age of the athletes, etc. Furthermore, estimations are complicated by under-reporting of the injury. Since a concussion cannot be "seen," athletes are able to conceal it from athletic trainers, team physicians, coaches, and parents. And many of them do. A 2004 study of high school American football players revealed that less than half of those sustaining a concussion reported it to anyone. Similar studies that have been conducted more than a decade later show similar results. Several reasons are given for this lack of reporting. Many younger athletes do not realize that they have sustained a concussion. Fewer realize that a concussion is a traumatic brain injury. They believe they have merely, "had their bell rung" or been "dinged." Even athletes who are knocked unconscious at the time of their injury often do not realize that they have sustained a concussion. In one medical study, high school athletes were allowed to write freely at the end of their questionnaires. One athlete recalled being sent to the athletic director after being knocked unconscious in order to see if he had a concussion. His interpretation after the meeting was that he did not have a concussion, despite the fact that he was knocked unconscious. He was free to return to sports. As athletes become older and more competitive, their reasons for under-reporting change. Many become afraid that reporting the injury jeopardizes their chance to keep their position on the team. Many are afraid that if they report their concussion, it will jeopardize their chance to play at a higher level. Some are seeking a chance to play in college. College athletes may be trying to go professional. Even professional athletes have been recorded as saying they did not want to report their concussion because they were afraid they would lose their starting position to a backup player. Either way, this under-reporting makes accurate estimations of injury difficult.

Furthermore, how commonly an injury occurs can be measured in a variety of ways. It can be measured as the number of players who sustain a concussion during a season. This fails to account for the number of athletes who are participating in a given sport or athletes who receive minimal or no play time. Furthermore, the rates of concussion are higher during competition than they are during practice. Sports like American football have relatively few games per season when compared to basketball or ice hockey. Measuring the numbers of concussions occurring per season does not take into account the number of competitions per season. In addition, some athletes will sustain multiple concussions during a single season. Measuring only the percentage of athletes who sustain a concussion during a season does not take into account those who sustain multiple concussions. In order to address these inaccuracies, some investigators have measured the number of concussions occurring for every "athletic exposure," where each practice and each competition count as one "athletic exposure." Others measure how many athletes will sustain a concussion out of every 100,000 athletes playing a given sport. Still others measure the percentage of total injuries during a season accounted for by concussions.

Studies have consistently demonstrated that, with the exception of cheerleading, concussions are more likely to occur during competition than during practice. This makes sense, as competitions are usually more intense and played more ferociously than practices. Taken all together, it is estimated that as many as 3.8 million sport-related traumatic brain injuries occur each year. The vast majority of these injuries are concussions. Cheerleading is thought to be an exception, as by the time competition comes around, cheerleaders are only executing stunts with which they have grade proficiency. Practice is the time when they are learning new stunts and therefore, perhaps, at greater risk of concussion.

Concussions account for between 9 and 13 percent of all organized athletic injuries in US high schools. Among pediatric patients, 30 to 50 percent of all concussions seen in United States emergency departments occur during sports. In United States colleges, concussions represent 6 percent of all organized athletic injuries. Approximately 20 percent of concussions that involve a loss of consciousness occur during sports and recreation.

American Football

American football is a fast-moving, hard-hitting, exciting game, watched by millions of Americans each week during the autumn. Given its popularity, it is one of the most frequently played sports by younger athletes. The recent retirement of some high-level professionals after sustaining multiple concussions has resulted in a lot of media attention about the rate of sport-related concussions in American football.

Approximately 1.8 million total athletes participate in American football annually, including 1.5 million high school athletes. Given the large numbers of athletes participating in it, American football accounts for the majority of the concussions that occur during team sports. In fact, some studies suggest that more than half of all sport-related concussions occurring in organized high school sports occur during football. Other studies suggest that 4 to 5 percent of high school and college football players will sustain a concussion during each season. Many of these studies, however, considered only those injuries diagnosed by the team's athletic trainer. As mentioned earlier, many athletes do not report their concussions. Interestingly, studies in which players have been asked directly and confidentially to report their symptoms after sustaining a blow to the head have revealed much higher rates of concussion, ranging from 15 to 45 percent of players per season.

Given the high rates of concussion in American football, in addition to the large number of athletes participating in it, efforts are being made to try and reduce the number of sport-related concussions that occur during American football. These efforts consist of rule changes, technical modifications to football helmets, changes in strength and conditioning, and stricter more consistent rule enforcement. These efforts have been inspired by former football players or the loved ones of former football players, who have suffered the effects of multiple concussions. Many readers may know the story of Christopher Nowinski, a former college football player from Harvard University and former professional wrestler who was forced to retire after sustaining multiple concussions that led to long-term problems. He is the author of the book *Mind Games: The NFL's Concussion Crisis*, a book I read when I first started learning about this issue.

ICE HOCKEY

Several studies suggest that ice hockey carries a higher risk of concussion than American football. Other studies suggest the rates are comparable. Still others suggest American football has a slightly higher incidence of concussion. Although the possibility that the incidence of concussion in ice hockey is higher than that of football surprises many people, studies that directly compare the two sports suggest that concussions are more common in ice hockey than in American football. The percentage of ice hockey players who sustain a concussion in a given season is higher than the percentage of American football players who sustain a concussion in a given season. A medical review of concussion in contact and collision sports, which included American football, ice hockey, rugby, and soccer, revealed that, for high school male athletes, ice hockey had the highest rates of concussion.

BASEBALL AND SOFTBALL

Approximately 720,000 high school athletes compete in baseball and softball per year. Concussion accounts for 3 to 6 percent of all injuries occurring during baseball and softball. However, the way in which baseball players sustain concussions differs from that of softball players. In baseball, concussions most often occur when the player is struck in the head with the ball. Catchers are at particular risk as they also sustain concussions during collisions at home plate with an oncoming base runner. Usually, the player is struck in the head with a pitch. In softball, however, while about half of concussions occur when the player is struck in the head with the ball, the remaining half are due to player-to-player collisions, collisions between a player and the outfield wall, or when the player's head strikes the ground after a fall.

BASKETBALL

Basketball is one of several sports that are popular with both boys and girls, men and women. As such, it gives us a unique insight into the effects gender might have on the rates of concussion. In girls' basketball, concussion accounts for 5 to 8 percent of all injuries, while in boys' basketball, it accounts for about

4 percent of all injuries. Some studies have suggested that high school girls who play basketball have a higher risk of concussion than high school boys who play basketball.

SOCCER

Soccer is also popular among male and female athletes. Again, this dual popularity in the similarity of the rules for both boys and girls allows us to compare the rates of concussions between boys and girls who play soccer. Much like basketball, studies that compare the number of concussions that occur in girls' soccer to the number of concussions that occur in boys' soccer suggest that girls may be at higher risk.

Overall, head injuries account for somewhere between 4 and 20 percent of all injuries in soccer. The goalkeeper seems to be at an increased risk of concussion when compared to other players. However, as noted earlier, athletes are often reluctant to report their concussion, which makes estimations of the rates of concussion difficult.

Some authors have suggested that the rates of concussion in soccer are similar to those in American football. However, this seems unlikely. These results are often cited by those who are comparing one medical study conducted in soccer players to a separate medical study conducted in football players. When one conducts a medical study in different populations, using different methods, it is ill-advised to compare the conclusions. Medical studies that used the same methods and same populations to compare the number of concussions occurring in soccer, American football, and several other sports reveal that concussion occurs more commonly during American football than during soccer.

When discussing sport-related concussion, soccer deserves some extra attention. The sport of soccer is unique in that players use their heads to advance the ball, pass to their teammates, and shoot on goal. This has led to speculation that concussion in soccer occurs from purposeful heading of the ball. Some studies have revealed poorer brain function in former soccer players than the general population. In particular, soccer players who report that they used to head the ball more often than their teammates had poorer brain function later in life than those former players who reported they purposefully headed the ball less often. Such studies have further fueled the speculation that purposeful heading of the ball causes concussions.

Several other studies, however, refute such a conclusion. In one such study, soccer players had their brain function measured before and after a soccer practice, which included 20 minutes of a dedicated heading exercise. No changes in brain function were noted. Since concussion often results in a decrease in brain function, the authors conclude purposeful heading does not cause concussions. Other studies have documented all of the concussions that were sustained over the course of a soccer tournament. Investigators reviewed how the concussions occurred by watching videotapes of the games. In such studies, no concussions occurred as a result of purposeful heading of the ball. Thus, many people feel concussions do not occur as a result of purposeful heading.

Since opening the Sports Concussion Clinic in the Division of Sports Medicine at Children's Hospital Boston in November 2008, we have cared for thousands of patients with concussions. Only a few have reported sustaining their concussions from purposeful heading of the ball. All of them were children.

Therefore, based on the current existing published studies regarding the incidence of concussion as it is related to purposeful heading of the soccer ball, I believe that purposeful heading of the ball is unlikely to cause a sport-related concussion. If an adult or teenage athlete sees the ball coming, sets up, and appropriately heads the ball with proper technique, concussion is unlikely. I believe for children, however, it is possible to sustain a concussion from purposefully heading the ball. One can imagine a young child, perhaps new to soccer, who is still developing physical coordination, standing under a ball that was punted up high by the goal keeper, and delivering a poorly timed, uncoordinated blow. The ball may have more of an effect on the acceleration of the child's head than the child's head has on the acceleration of the ball. In this situation, I believe concussion is possible. The risk of this is likely increased if children are sent out to play with adult-size soccer balls, as opposed to smaller balls more suitable for their size.

Some have suggested that perhaps children should not be allowed to head the ball until they reach a certain age and have become stronger and better coordinated. In fact, the last several years the U.S. soccer has recommended no heading for players under the age of 10 and only limited amounts of heading during practice for those between the ages of 11 and 13. I can understand the emotions behind making such a recommendation; however, I think it is a mistake without at least teaching children the proper technique for having a ball at a younger age. As children become stronger and better coordinated, they are able to kick the ball at a much greater velocity. It seems unwise to have their first time trying to head a ball occur at an age when the ball can be kicked with significant speed and force. Instead, using smaller, softer balls that weigh less while children are younger would allow them to develop the skills necessary for proper heading of the ball. This seems like a safer approach. They can learn proper technique, develop strength, and master the timing and coordination necessary for proper heading of the ball when young, before the ball can be kicked with significant force. I received several phone calls from many sports medicine physicians, neurologists, and other doctors involved with coaching soccer asking what to do after this recommendation was made. It is always difficult to answer such a question as I don't want to be in the position of recommending something that goes against an existing rule. One possible alternative would be to teach the skills involved in heading a soccer ball by using a Nerf soccer ball or other similar soft balls in practice. This will allow young soccer players to learn proper technique without exposing them to the higher force collisions involved by using a regulation ball. I know of a neurologist who also coaches soccer and uses a balloon to teach such technique.

LACROSSE

First played by the Native Americans, lacrosse is a sport growing in popularity in the United States. For the reader unfamiliar with it, lacrosse has rules similar to ice hockey, but it is played on grass or turf. Players carry a stick with a net on the end of it. The net is used to carry the lacrosse ball. In order to score, the ball has to be thrown into the opponent's net, past the goalkeeper. Boys' and men's lacrosse are collision sports, where players are allowed to collide body to body, and defending players are allowed to use their sticks to strike at the offending player who is carrying the ball, in order to free the ball from his possession. According to the rules of women's lacrosse, such contact is not allowed.

Although fewer people play lacrosse when compared to other sports, concussion rates in lacrosse are fairly high. As in most collision sports, concussions in lacrosse most often occur during body to body collisions with an opponent. But they also occur from collisions with the ground, and from being struck in the head with the ball.

RUGBY

As with many collision sports, concussion is common in rugby, accounting for about 16 percent of all injuries. It usually occurs secondary to body-to-body contact with another player. In one study, concussions accounted for 40 percent of all injuries that occurred during illegal or foul play. Unlike soccer and basketball, the risk of concussion in women's rugby is similar to that in men's.

SKIING AND SNOWBOARDING

Downhill skiing and snowboarding are popular sports in North America and Europe in which amateur participants travel at surprisingly high rates of speed, surrounded by snow, ice, trees, large metallic chair-lift poles, and fellow snow sport enthusiasts. Head injuries account for up to 20 percent of all injuries in these sports. Recently, some high-profile celebrities have sustained tragic head injuries, drawing much needed attention to the risks of these sports. When I was growing up in New England, the use of helmets while skiing was almost unheard of. Now, it is the norm.

In fact, I went skiing with a bunch of work colleagues several years ago. When we arrived at the ski slope, we took all of our equipment from the car and headed for the bottom of the chair lifts. Once I had my skis attached and my poles ready, I looked up and saw that I was the only one, in a group of five or six skiers, who was not wearing a helmet. In addition to calling me crazy, they laughed and joked about how it was ironic that the physician among us whose career was dedicated to caring for athletes who sustain head injuries in sports was the only one without a helmet. Until that point, it had never occurred to me to wear a helmet while skiing. Now, I wouldn't go downhill skiing without one.

As men and women both participate in these downhill sports, comparisons can be made between the sexes. Male skiers are nearly twice as likely to sustain a head injury as women skiers. Furthermore, concussions sustained by female skiers are more often due to collisions with another person, while those sustained by male skiers are more often a result of collisions with an object. Although the reasons for the difference in incidence of concussion between male and female skiers are unknown, there are several possibilities. It could be due to the amount of risk taken by male skiers. It may be that female skiers are wiser and more cautious whereas male skiers are little more reckless.

COMBAT SPORTS

Wrestling is a combat sport that does not allow for deliberate blows to the head by the opponent. Rather combatants try to control one another by placing their opponents in various holds. Concussion accounts for 4 to 5 percent of all injuries in wrestling. Nearly half of the concussions in wrestling are due to takedowns. A recent National Collegiate Athletic Association (NCAA) study suggested that among all collegiate sports, wrestling had the highest incidence of concussion, exceeding that of American football, men's ice hockey, and women's soccer. There are, however, many other studies suggesting that wrestling has a lower incidence of concussion than these sports.

Unlike wrestling, combat sports such as boxing allow for purposeful, direct blows to the head. Boxing is unique in that one of the main purposes of the competition is to concuss your opponent. If you deliver a blow to your opponent that knocks him unconscious for 10 seconds or longer, you win the bout. If you do not knock your opponent unconscious, but are able to concuss him such that he is dazed, confused, off-balance, or has a slower reaction time, your task of delivering further blows becomes easier, as he is less capable of defending himself. It is this nature of boxing that has made it so controversial, especially when it comes to children participating. Without entering into the controversy, I will simply say that concussion is a common occurrence in boxing. Perhaps more concerning, the possible effects of multiple blows to the head that do not result in concussion have been raised recently. This will be discussed further in Chapter 12.

Perhaps even more controversial than boxing, the popularity of mixed martial arts has risen dramatically over the last 20 years. Similar to boxing, mixed martial arts allows for blows to the head of one's opponent. Once again, the bout can be won by knocking the opponent unconscious, and significant advantage can be gained by concussing one's opponent, even if he is not knocked unconscious. Studies suggest that a concussion occurs in one out of every 10 mixed martial arts matches.

Cheerleading

Cheerleading has changed dramatically over the last 40 years. When I was a kid, cheerleaders literally led the cheers of the crowd. They organized and inspired the crowd. Occasionally, they might tumble, or do some handsprings. Nowadays, however, major cheerleading squads are more like a combination of gymnasts and acrobats. They perform stunts, often as high as 20 feet in the air, without the added precaution of pads or netting. They are thrown up in the air by other cheerleaders, and come crashing down into their colleagues' arms. Thus, it is not surprising that the rates of concussions occurring in cheerleaders have risen dramatically. Cheerleading has the unique distinction of being one of the only sports in which concussion is more common during practice than competition. As might be expected, more than 90 percent of concussions in cheerleading occur during a stunt.

A note of caution is warranted. As can be seen from some of the previous summaries, medical studies are not always consistent. The incidence of injury varies from study to study, and the relative incidence of concussion between sports varies by study. Therefore, clinicians and researchers rarely base their opinion on a single medical study. More often, we try to read the vast majority of studies conducted on a given topic and use the entirety of the published evidence when forming an opinion.

Should Children Participate in These Sports?

Chapter 10 will discuss this question in greater detail, but it warrants some mentioning here as well. In order to practice medicine, one must continuously weigh the potential risks of a given action against its known or potential benefits. While concussion is a risk in nearly all sports, the benefits from sports participation and athletic competition are innumerable. For children, sports participation increases their physical health, cardiovascular conditioning, strength, and endurance. It improves their self-image. It decreases the risk of obesity. It decreases the risk of incarceration, illegal drug use, teen pregnancy, and sexually transmitted diseases. It increases future academic and career success. By preparing for competition, children learn that they can improve their performance and skills through practice and hard work. Those children engaged in team sports learn to interact with their peers, to assist those who are less skilled, and to learn from those who are more highly skilled. They learn to cooperate. They learn to lead.

Furthermore, we in America are in the midst of an obesity epidemic fueled by physical inactivity. The rates of obesity in U.S. children have quadrupled in the last 30 years due, in part, to decreased levels of physical activity. The Centers for Disease Control and Prevention and the Surgeon General have issued recommendations aimed at decreasing obesity and increasing physical activity. Medical studies have shown that regular bouts of physical activity in childhood lead to more active lifestyles in adulthood. For adults, sports participation increases strength, endurance, cardiovascular conditioning, mood, and energy levels and improves self-image. It lowers cholesterol levels. It decreases the risk of heart attack, stroke, obesity, depression. Exercise guarantees benefits. In fact, a person's individual, habitual amount of regular exercise is the most significant determinant of death from all causes.

Most athletes will recover completely from their injuries, including concussions. So, while we all should try to decrease the number of injuries sustained by athletes and treat athletic injuries appropriately when they occur, athletes should be encouraged to continue to participate in sports. Even after sustaining a concussion, athletes should be encouraged to return to their preferred sports, as long as it is medically safe to do so.

In summary, concussion is a risk in almost any sport. Combat and collision sports carry a higher risk of concussion than contact and noncontact sports. But the risks of concussion in contact sports, which do not involve purposeful collisions, are still significant. The risk of sustaining a sport-related concussion, however, is often outweighed by the tremendous benefits that athletes derive from participation in sports. Concussions, if managed properly, should not prevent athletes from engaging in those sports that they love. For a small minority of athletes who experience multiple concussions, or significant, prolonged, or incomplete recoveries from their concussions, sports participation may be restricted to certain safer sports and athletic activities.

SUGGESTED READINGS

Fuller, C. W., A. Junge, and J. Dvorak. A six year prospective study of the incidence and causes of head and neck injuries in international football. *Br J Sports Med*, 2005, 39 (Suppl 1): p. i3–i9.

Gerberich, S. G., et al. Concussion incidences and severity in secondary school varsity football players. *Am J Public Health*, 1983, 73(12): 1370–1375.

Hainline, B., and R. G. Ellenbogen. A perfect storm. *J Athl Train*, 2017, 52 (3): 157–159.

Koh, J.O., J. D. Cassidy, and E. J. Watkinson. Incidence of concussion in contact sports: A systematic review of the evidence. *Brain Inj*, 2003, 17(10): 901–917.

MacDonald, J., and G. D. Myer. "Don't let kids play football": A killer idea. *Br J Sports Med*, October 8, 2016 [Epub ahead of print].

Nonfatal traumatic brain injuries from sports and recreation activities—United States, 2001–2005. *Morb Mortal Wkly Rep*, 2007, 56(29): 733–737.

Nowinski, C. *Head Games: Football's Concussion Crisis*. East Bridgewater, MA: The Drummond Publishing Group, 2007.

Shulz, M.R., et al. Incidence and risk factors for concussion in high school athletes, North Carolina, 1996–1999. *Am J Epidemiol,* 2004, 160: 937–944.

Zuckerman, S. L., Z. Y. Kerr, A. Yengo-Kahn, E. Wasserman, T. Covassin, and G. S. Solomon. Epidemiology of sports-related concussion in NCAA athletes from 2009–2010 to 2013–2014: Incidence, recurrence, and mechanisms. *Am J Sports Med,* 2015, 43(11): 2654–2662.

3

Risk Factors for Concussion: What Factors Are Associated with an Increased Risk of Sustaining a Concussion or Suffering a Long Recovery?

On December 12, 2015, in a fight that was preceded by substantial amounts of trash talk, Conor McGregor fought Jose Aldo for the UFC featherweight title. Both men emerged from their corners with a lot of energy to begin the fight. Ten seconds into the fight, Jose Aldo lunged at McGregor and swung a left hook towards McGregor's head. But as he did, McGregor slipped a left cross straight to the jaw of Jose Aldo, knocking him unconscious. Only 13 seconds into the fight, Jose Aldo was concussed, and Conor McGregor was the new champion. It was the shortest title fight and UFC history.

In medicine, we often discuss risk factors for a certain disease, injury, or medical condition. A risk factor is some characteristic, physical attributes, environmental exposure, or other factor that is associated with an increased risk of developing a disease, sustaining an injury, or suffering from a certain medical condition. One common example of a risk factor that is associated with disease is cigarette smoking. Cigarette smoking is a strong risk factor for lung cancer, meaning those who smoke cigarettes regularly are much at higher risk of developing lung cancer than those individuals who have never smoked. In addition, smoking increases the risk of heart disease and several other medical conditions. Obesity and high cholesterol levels are examples of risk factors for heart disease and for suffering a heart attack.

Risk factors come in two main forms: modifiable and not modifiable. The examples noted earlier are modifiable risk factors. One could stop smoking cigarettes and thereby decrease the risk of developing lung cancer that is associated with cigarette smoking. In fact, avoidance entirely of cigarette smoking is the best way of decreasing the risk of lung cancer. Similarly, overweight people that have high cholesterol can reduce the risk of heart disease by losing weight and by decreasing their cholesterol levels by changing their diet, exercising more regularly, and taking medications that decrease their cholesterol levels. These are all examples of modifiable risk factors, those risk factors that can be adjusted.

Some risk factors are not modifiable. For example, having a strong family history of heart disease is also a risk factor for heart disease. One is not able to modify his or her family history. If your father and grandfather both suffered heart attacks at a young age, there is nothing you can do to change that fact. Therefore, that risk factor is not modifiable. There are risk factors that are associated with increased incidence of sport-related concussion. "Incidence" is a word that describes the occurrence or frequency of a disease injury or medical condition. In the example of sport-related concussion, we often measure the incidence of concussions, meaning the number of concussions that occur over the course of a given sport season or year. In fact, a preferable way of measuring the incidence of concussions in sports is the number of concussions that occur per athletic exposure. As discussed in Chapter 2, an athletic exposure is defined as one athlete participating in one practice or one competition. For example, a soccer team that consists of 30 players and practices four days a week would have 30 athletic exposures per day, or 120 athletic exposures per week. Measuring the incidence of concussion this way allows us to compare across sports the risk of concussion. For example, if the risk of suffering a sport-related concussion was 7 concussions per 10,000 athletic exposures in American football and 4 concussions per 10,000 athletic exposures in men's lacrosse, we would say that football is associated with an increased incidence of concussion compared to men's lacrosse.

There are several risk factors that are associated with an increased incidence of concussion. Some are modifiable and some are not modifiable. In the example noted earlier, sports would be considered a risk factor for sport-related concussion. One can imagine without even reviewing the medical literature that the incidence of sport-related concussion in sports such as American football, rugby, men's ice hockey, and men's lacrosse, sports where purposeful body to body collisions or frank tackling is allowed, is higher than the incidence of sport-related concussion in sports where there is no body-to-body contact such as tennis, golf, swimming, and cross-country running. Therefore, perhaps the largest modifiable risk factor for sport-related concussion is the sport in which the athlete is participating. If an athlete wishes to decrease the risk of sustaining a sport-related concussion, they could modify the sports in which they participate such that they participate in sports with a lower risk of concussion. An athlete who is concerned about the risk of sport-related concussion that is associated with ice hockey, for example, could switch his or her winter sport to basketball, which has a lower incidence of sport-related concussion, or even swimming, which has a much lower risk of sport-related concussion.

Many athletes, however, would find it unacceptable to switch their sport. Athletes often play certain sports because they enjoy those sports more than the other options offered during the same season. Furthermore, athletes usually enjoy sports to which they can make a meaningful contribution more than those to which they are unable to contribute meaningfully to the overall effort of the team. Therefore, an athlete who is particularly good at football, say, may be less inclined to participate in cross-country if he is not able to stand long periods of fast running. As such, we often look for other risk factors that are modifiable rather than recommending an athlete switch his or her preferred sport.

There are certain positions within sports that are associated with an increased incidence of concussion. For example, many athletes participate in baseball. Baseball is fortunate to be a sport in which the incidence of concussion is lower than many other team sports. Even within sports, however, the incidence of concussion varies between the positions. Catchers, for example, appear to be at an increased risk of sport-related concussion compared to other positions in baseball. Therefore, athletes who enjoy participating in baseball but are worried about the incidence of concussion or the potential of sustaining a concussion might consider switching their position from catcher to say, third base.

Certain types of play are also associated with an increased risk of concussion. For example, body checking men's ice hockey is associated with increased risk of concussion. By removing body check in ice hockey, through a changing of the rules, one could potentially reduce the incidence of concussion. The same may be said of tackle football. It is quite possible that if one were to eliminate tackling from football and turn it into touch football or flag football, the incidence of concussion might decrease. While this may seem obvious to certain readers, it is worth noting that in a prospective study of injuries in youth football, the incidence of injury was higher in flag football than it was in tackle football. There was no significant difference between the incidence of severe injuries or concussions between tackle football and flag football. This study underscores one important point of doing research: our assumptions are not always correct, even when they seem obvious.

Similarly, while purposeful heading of the soccer ball does not in and of itself usually result in a concussion, the act of heading is high risk, as there is usually an opponent also making a play for the ball. Many concussions occur not because of purposeful heading of the ball, but rather, when the athlete's struck by another athlete who is making an attempt to get the ball during the act of purposefully heading the ball, or gets tangled up with another athlete and falls striking the head on the ground. Therefore, by limiting purposeful heading of the ball during soccer, one would likely reduce the incidence of sport-related concussion.

All of these hypothetical rule changes, however, would dramatically change the way the game is played. For some athletes, the change in the game may be welcomed, especially if it is associated with a decreased risk of concussion. For others, however, part of their love of the game may come from purposefully heading a soccer ball or from the physicality involved with tackling in football or body checking in ice hockey. It could be that for these athletes to make a meaningful contribution to the team their size and strength and ability to generate power are important. If tackling or body checking was removed from the game, their importance to the team might drop. They might become less interested in participating. Therefore, when making such rule changes, one must weigh the benefits of reduction in sport-related injuries against the changes to the game. One option would be to allow both forms of the games, such that one could expand non-tackling football leagues as well as expand non-checking ice hockey leagues for those who wish to play those sports but do not wish to be involved in the physical nature of them as currently played.

Collision anticipation is also a risk factor associated with sport-related concussion. When athletes see collisions coming, they instinctively brace for the oncoming collision, prepare their body in an athletic stance, and often drive through the collision, thereby decreasing their risk of injury. Evidence generated by studying the concussions that occur during sports has shown that inadequate collision anticipation that does not allow enough for the athlete to prepare his or her body for impact his associated with an increased incidence of concussion compared to collisions that occur after sufficient time for proper anticipation. Therefore, coaching strategies to help athletes anticipate and prepare their bodies for collisions might result in a decreased incidence of concussion. Collision anticipation is thus, at least somewhat, a modifiable risk factor.

Neck strength is also likely a modifiable risk factor for sport-related concussion. Please recall from Chapter 1 of this book that concussion is due to a rapid rotation of the brain. For a given force, the resulting acceleration of the head after collision is inversely proportional to the mass. That is to say, the greater mass of the head that sustains a collision, the lower the acceleration after the collision. Since one increases the effective mass of the head by attaching it rigidly to the body, therefore causing the head and the body to act as one unit, one might reduce the resulting acceleration of the head after a collision. Since it is this acceleration that results in concussion, one might be able to reduce the incidence of concussion. Since the head is attached to the remainder of the body by the muscles of the neck, the stronger the neck muscles are, the more effectively than might attach it to the body, thereby potentially reducing the incidence of concussion. This type of thinking has led to the hypothesis that greater neck strength is associated with a decreased risk of concussion. Indeed, there have been several studies that suggest that athletes with stronger neck muscles have a lower incidence of concussion than athletes with weaker necks. Since one can strengthen the muscles of the neck through resistance training, neck strength is a modifiable risk factor for concussion. Specifically, what are known as isometric exercises, those in which the athlete generates force using the muscles of the neck without actually moving the head, can be performed safely in conjunction with a certified strength and conditioning specialist or other responsible adult in order to increase the strength of the muscles of the neck, potentially decreasing the incidence of concussion.

Lastly, it is possible that certain types of equipment are associated with an increased or decreased incidence of concussion. This can be field equipment from the field of play or personal equipment that an athlete wears on his or her body. One can imagine that striking one's head against a hard metal goalpost could result in a sport-related concussion. By providing a thick, foam padding around the goalpost that will slowly collapse and slow the speed of an oncoming athlete, one might decrease the incidence of concussion. Thus, the equipment used on the field might represent a modifiable risk factor for sport-related concussion.

Personal equipment might also be associated with the risk of concussion. One can imagine a different type of helmet, mouth guard, shoulder pad, or other forms of equipment might be associated with an increased or decreased risk of concussion. As of yet, since most equipment was designed to reduce the risk of other injuries, the evidence is inconclusive as to whether these personal equipment items can be modified in such a way to significantly reduce the incidence of concussion. This will be discussed in greater detail in the next chapter. Personal equipment does represent, however, a potential opportunity for decreasing the risk of concussion.

There are, of course, of non-modifiable risk factors associated with the incidence of concussion as well. Some studies suggest that for a given sport in which the rules are similar between male and female participants, the incidence of concussion may be higher among female athletes. There are several research investigations that support this claim. Studies remain inconclusive, however, as the incidence of injury is often determined by self-report; there may be other factors associated with reporting of injuries between women and men that explain part of this finding. It could be that simply girls are more likely to report their injuries than boys are and, therefore, while the incidence might be similar between boys and girls, it appears greater for girls as they are reporting more of their injuries. Either way sex is not a modifiable risk factor. (I do, recognize, that there are transgender persons and persons who have undergone sex change operations participating in sports. I am aware of no evidence, however, that being transgender or having a sex changing operation is associated with an increased or decreased risk of sport-related concussion.)

Similarly there may be biological characteristics that are associated with an increased or decreased risk of concussion. There may be genetic predisposition to concussion. Genetic makeup represents a non-modifiable risk factor for concussion. In addition, anatomy, the way the brain is shaped or sits within the skull, might also be associated with an increased or decreased risk of sport-related concussion. There are several studies investigating these possibilities, but at present it remains largely unknown whether genetic makeup or anatomical considerations are associated with the risk of sport-related concussion.

In addition to incidence, there are risk factors associated with a long recovery after a concussion occurs. Some of these are modifiable, and some are not modifiable. For example, there have been studies suggesting that an athlete who sustains a concussion but continues to participate in sport might suffer a longer recovery than those who recognized the injury and removed themselves from play immediately. By educating athletes as to the signs and symptoms of concussion and the potential downside of continuing to play through concussion, we could modify this risk factor, resulting in increased recognition of injuries and an increased removal from play.

Some risk factors are not modifiable. Several studies suggest that athletes who have sustained multiple concussions, on average, require longer periods of time to recover than those who have sustained their first lifetime concussion. This is particularly true if the previous concussions occur within a short time frame, especially within the previous year. The number of concussions an athlete has sustained previously is not however modifiable. Furthermore, there is evidence that sex (male or female) is also associated with an increased duration of symptoms after a concussion occurs. Again sex is not easily modified and would be considered mostly a non-modifiable risk factor. Finally, certain preexisting medical conditions are associated with prolonged recovery from sport-related concussion. In particular, learning disabilities and attention deficit hyperactivity disorder are often associated with longer recovery after sport-related concussion.

In summary, there are several established and several possible risk factors associated with the incidence of concussion. There are also several established and several possible risk factors associated with a prolonged recovery from concussion. Some of these are modifiable, while others are not. The most common modifiable risk factors include sport, position within a given sport, certain behaviors or styles of play, the ability to anticipate collisions, the type of equipment used, and the response to sport-related concussion when it occurs. Efforts to prevent sport-related concussions focus on modifiable risk factors.

SUGGESTED READINGS

Green, G. A., K. M. Pollack, J. D'Angelo, M. S. Schickendantz, R. Caplinger, K. Weber, A. Valadka, T. W. McAllister, R. W. Dick, B. Mandelbaum, and F. C. Curriero. Mild traumatic brain injury in major and Minor League Baseball players. *Am J Sports Med*, 2015, 43(5): 1118–1126.

Iverson, G. L., et al. Predictors of clinical recovery from concussion: A systematic review. *Br J Sports Med*, 2017, 51(12): 941–948.

Mihalik, J. P., et al. Collision type and player anticipation affect head impact severity among youth ice hockey players. *Pediatrics*, 2010, 125(6): e1394–e401.

Peterson, A. R., A. J. Kruse, S. M. Meester, T. S. Olson, B. N. Riedle, T. G. Slayman, T. J. Domeyer, J. E. Cavanaugh, and M. K. Smoot. Youth football injuries: A prospective cohort. *Orthop J Sports Med*, 2017, 5(2): 2325967116686784.

Roberts, W. O., et al. Fair-play rules and injury reduction and ice hockey. *Arch Pediatr Adolesc Med*, 1996, 150(2): 140–145.

4

SPORTS EQUIPMENT: HELMETS, MOUTH GUARDS, AND CONCUSSION PREVENTION

On October 3, 2010, the New York Giants dominated the Chicago Bears. The Giants defense seemed nearly unstoppable in the first half, tallying nine sacks of the Bears' quarterback, Jay Cutler. On the second to last play of the half, Giants cornerback, number 31, Aaron Ross, raced in unopposed from Cutler's left side. With the Bears quarterback secured within his grasp, Ross spun Cutler around 180 degrees and hurled him to the ground. The left side of Cutler's helmet, securely fastened to his head, bounced off of the ground sharply. Cutler was hesitant to get up. He was removed from the game.

Jay Cutler was concussed.

This chapter will discuss the potential role of personal protective gear in reducing the risk of concussions. The medical evidence regarding helmets, mouth guards, and other such protective equipment often advertised as capable of reducing concussion will be discussed.

Many people believe that football players wear helmets in order to reduce their risk of concussion. In fact, helmets were not designed for this purpose. Prior to the use of the modern-day helmets, catastrophic brain injuries, such as bleeding into the brain and massive swelling of the brain, used to occur at unacceptably high rates. Helmets were invented to reduce these catastrophic brain injuries, a task at which they are highly effective. But, it is likely that athletes wearing helmets play more aggressively than those without helmets. As a result, the introduction of helmets to a sport is more likely to increase the risk of concussion than to decrease it. In fact, changes to more aggressive behaviors within a sport in response to the introduction of protective equipment have been noted in men's ice hockey, equestrian, cycling, and other activities. Since helmets reduce the risk of death and devastating neurological outcomes after head injury, most people believe that the increased risk of concussion is a price worth paying.

Many companies advertise protective equipment by claiming it can reduce the risk of concussion. Companies selling helmets, mouth guards, headbands, "custom mandibular orthotics," and various other devices make such claims on their packaging, websites, and in advertisements. Yet the Centers for Disease Control and Prevention, American Academy of Pediatrics, and experts on concussion in sports contend that there is no equipment available that has been proven to reduce the risk of concussion. In fact, there have been Congressional hearings regarding the false advertising claims made by equipment manufacturers with regard to their ability to decrease the incidence of concussion. As a result, many athletes, coaches, and parents are confused by the mixed messages. Here, we will discuss the reasons for the two separate messages and review the available medical evidence regarding these devices.

In the early 1900s, American football was recognized as a dangerous sport. An offensive formation known as "the flying wedge" often led to significant injuries. In 1905, concerned by the number of deaths and catastrophic injuries sustained by American football players, President Theodore Roosevelt summoned college athletic directors to the White House for a meeting. This group of athletic leaders, led by New York University Chancellor Henry Mac-Cracken, formed the group that ultimately grew to call itself the National Collegiate Athletic Association (NCAA). One of the main functions of the NCAA was, and remains to this day, to set the rules and regulations for intercollegiate American football and other sports.

However, it may surprise readers to know that football helmets were brought about by players, as opposed to rules set by the NCAA or other athletic organizations. Initially, the football helmet was nothing more than a leather hat and strap. The main intention was to prevent cauliflower ear, and perhaps, offer some protection to the head. Early versions of the modern-day plastic helmet did not appear until the 1930s. The helmet itself did not become mandatory in the National Football League until the 1940s. It may further surprise readers to learn that engineers designing the football helmet were not trying to prevent concussion. Back when the modern-day football helmet was being designed, catastrophic injuries to the brain such as swelling of the brain, bleeding into or around the brain, skull fractures and death were much more common than they are today. The goal of these early helmets was to prevent these catastrophic injuries, which often resulted in death, coma, or neurological devastation. At the time, concussive brain injury was poorly understood. Most people, including physicians, did not recognize it as a significant injury. Therefore, there was no effort to try to prevent concussions, or to try and design helmets that could prevent concussion.

Only recently has the medical community realized that concussion results in true brain dysfunction. For this, and several other reasons discussed in this book, there is a renewed interest in trying to prevent concussions.

As stated earlier, some companies advertise protective equipment for reducing the risk of concussions. Yet many, if not most, medical experts maintain there is no such protective device available. This discrepancy likely results from differing interpretations of the available medical research data. We will review the available data here.

FOOTBALL HELMETS

As noted earlier, football helmets were not originally designed to prevent concussions or even reduce the risk of concussion. They were designed to prevent catastrophic brain injury, death, or severe neurological injury. Despite that, there have been some studies examining the risk of concussions for athletes wearing various helmets. One such study suggested a slightly lower risk of concussion for athletes using a particular helmet. This led many to think that this helmet decreased the risk of sustaining a concussion while playing football. However, the methods and statistical analyses used to conduct this research left the conclusions vulnerable to doubt. Other studies have not been able to confirm these conclusions. Therefore, there is no convincing data demonstrating the ability of any given available helmet to decrease an athlete's risk of concussion.

One additional medical study investigated the rates of concussion in athletes wearing more modern types of helmets and compared them to the rates of concussion in athletes wearing older types of helmets made with previous technology. Their results seemed to suggest that the new type of helmet technology may reduce the risk of sport-related concussions, at least in American football. However, the study has been criticized for failing to account for all other possible factors. Those wearing the helmets with the newer technology were also wearing newer helmets. Those athletes wearing helmets made using older technology were wearing older helmets, helmets that have seen more play time and thus suffered significantly more wear and tear. It could be that the perceived benefit was not, in fact, due to the new helmet technology, but rather due to the fact that the helmets were new, and therefore, in peak condition.

Only in the last few years have engineers been designing helmets with the specific intention of reducing the risks of concussion. While this new effort is encouraging, at the time of this writing, there has been little, convincing, published data on the effects of these newer helmet technologies. It is uncertain whether it will, in fact, reduce the risks of an athlete sustaining a concussion.

ICE HOCKEY HELMETS

The risks of head injury, cervical spine injury, and concussion in ice hockey are higher than most other team sports. These athletes are in a unique situation. They are on ice, a hard, slippery surface, on which it is difficult to balance. They are wearing skates, which force them to balance their bodies on a thin, sleek, metallic blade. They are constantly colliding with one another in an attempt to knock each other off balance, off the puck, or out of the play. They are surrounded by hard dasher boards and Plexiglas. And they are capable of reaching high levels of speed, at times, exceeding 30 miles per hour. This is a setup for head and neck injuries. Thus, mandating the use of helmets in ice hockey is an obvious result. In order to reduce the risk of catastrophic head injuries, all ice hockey players should wear an undamaged, properly fitted helmet with the chin strap affixed appropriately. Players, however, should know that these helmets will not reduce the risk of concussion. Playing with the head up, being aware of other players and objects around you, anticipating oncoming collisions, and being in peak condition are still the most effective defenses against sport-related concussions in ice hockey.

BICYCLE HELMETS

Perhaps the biggest impact helmets have made on athlete safety is in the realm of bicycling. Medical studies have demonstrated a decreased number of deaths in various populations since the introduction of bicycle helmet legislation. Unfortunately, for many of the same reasons discussed earlier in other sports, bicycle helmets do not definitively reduce the risk of concussion. In fact, some medical researchers feel that cyclists wearing bicycle helmets take more risks than those without helmets. Thus, while the risk of death and catastrophic brain injury may be decreased by wearing a helmet, the rates of concussion may in fact increase. Either way, given their well-established ability to reduce the risk of death and catastrophic injury, cyclists should wear helmets.

I sold my car when my wife and I got married. Since then, I bike to work, to the store, to meet with friends, almost everywhere. I always wear my helmet. In addition, the employees of the Division of Sports Medicine at Children's Hospital Boston used to hold weekend bike rides together. I have never seen one of the members of our division cycling without a helmet.

SKIING AND SNOWBOARDING HELMETS

There is some evidence that helmets may reduce the risk of concussion in these alpine sports. There is good medical evidence that wearing helmets while skiing or snowboarding will reduce the risk of head injuries. A study involving over 20,000 skiers and snow boarders concluded that those wearing helmets had a 15 percent decreased risk of sustaining a head injury after a fall or collision compared to skiers and snowboarders not wearing a helmet. Please note that this study measured the risk of all head injuries, not specifically concussion.

Why helmets might help reduce the risk of concussion in one sport but not in others remains unclear. It could result from changes in behavior on the part of athletes. It is thought by some doctors and other medical researchers that in contact and collision sports such as football and ice hockey, there is a general respect for the head. Few, if any, athletes hope to cause harm or injure another athlete. Some have speculated that athletes who are not wearing helmets during these high-risk sports show some restraint when delivering a blow to one of their opponents. However, when athletes are covered in helmets and other forms of padding, there may be a sense of indestructibility. Therefore, athletes who are playing fully padded are more likely to deliver and receive more aggressive and forceful blows than those who are not so effectively padded. Since, in general, the helmets and pads do not significantly reduce the rotational acceleration of the head after impact, they have no effect on the risk of sport-related concussion. In skiing and snowboarding, however, concussion seldom results from a purposeful blow. Rather, concussive brain injury results from an accident in which the skier strikes a tree, the mountain, or other inanimate object. On occasion, it may occur from two skiers or snowboarders colliding. Since these injuries do not result from purposeful collisions, they are less likely to be affected by changes in behavior or attitude.

This is, however, speculation. Other investigators have argued that, even in sports such as skiing or bicycling where purposeful blows are not delivered to one's opponents, wearing helmets increases the risk of concussive brain injury. These medical investigators hypothesize that athletes wearing helmets while participating in these sports engage in more risk-taking behavior. For example, they argue that cyclists wearing helmets travel at higher speeds, ride on more rugged terrain, dart in and out of traffic more readily, and are less likely to obey the rules of traffic. There is some medical evidence to support both sides of this argument. It seems likely, given the current available medical evidence, that modern-day helmets do not significantly decrease the risk of an athlete sustaining a sport-related concussion. In fact, they may increase the risk to some unknown degree.

IMPORTANT NOTE TO THE READER: While today's helmets may not be effective in preventing concussion, they are highly effective at preventing catastrophic brain injury. Therefore, all athletes participating in high-risk activities should wear a new, undamaged, properly fitted helmet.

MOUTH GUARDS

Mouth guards have been cited by some as potentially preventing concussive brain injury. Several such studies were performed in cadavers, the bodies of dead people. As readers of this book have already learned, the concussed brain is not structurally damaged; it is not significantly swollen, bruised, bleeding, or otherwise damaged. Concussion is a problem with brain function. The concussed brain does not work properly. Concussed patients have poor memory, poor concentration, headaches, difficulty sleeping, trouble with balance, etc. Since brain function cannot be assessed in a cadaver, we can draw minimal conclusion about the effects of preventing concussion from studies using cadavers.

Other studies have been performed in living athletes, both to determine whether concussions are less likely to occur in athletes wearing a mouth guard and whether those wearing a mouth guard have fewer symptoms, less-significant decreases in brain function, or faster recoveries.

In a study published in 2007 in the journal *Dental Traumatology*, Jason Mihalik and colleagues measured neurocognitive function in two groups of athletes: those who sustained a concussion while wearing a mouth guard and those who sustained a concussion while not wearing a mouth guard. They found no differences in brain function between the two groups, meaning mouth guards did not prevent a loss of brain function after concussive brain injury.

In a 1987 study of rugby players published in the *British Journal of Sports Medicine*, Blignault and colleagues showed no statistical difference in the rates of concussion between rugby players wearing mouth guards and those not wearing mouth guards.

More recent studies have claimed that custom-made, form-fitting, special individualized mouth guards called custom mandibular orthotics (CMOs) may decrease the rates of concussion. However, the results are unclear. The methods used to conduct the research were poor, leading to unreliable and perhaps frankly erroneous conclusions. Therefore, no definitive conclusions can be drawn. Any effects of CMOs and other mouth guards on concussions remains unknown.

As with helmets, however, it is well-established that mouth guards reduce the risk of facial bone fractures and dental injuries. Therefore, all athletes participating in sports that require the use of a mouth guard should wear an undamaged, properly fitting mouth guard while they are playing.

Soccer Headbands

More recently, soccer players, coaches, and parents of soccer players have been asking about the ability of headbands to reduce the risk of concussion. Indeed, many headbands advertise such an ability. There is little medical evidence to support this assertion.

In a study published in the *British Journal of Sports Medicine* in 2000, McIntosh and McCrory studied eight commercially available head protectors designed for soccer players. They measured the ability of these protective devices to reduce energy at impact. They further investigated how well these devices maintained their function over time, after repeated impacts. As might be expected, they concluded that protective headgear for soccer players can reduce the risk of scalp lacerations, cuts, and abrasions, but that any reduction in the risk of sustaining a concussion is unlikely.

Other studies have suggested a potential benefit of soccer headgear in reducing the risk of concussion. So those of us caring for athletes cannot be certain as to whether these devices are effective. Certainly, medical studies showing a potential benefit and those not showing a benefit are limited. In some, there were other significant differences between the players wearing headgear and those not wearing headgear. In one study in particular, athletes who wore headgear were more likely to be female, to have suffered concussions previously and to wear a mouth guard. Given these differences, these athletes may have played more cautiously than those not wearing headgear. It could be their cautious play that seemed to reduce their risk of concussion. Perhaps, given their history of previous concussions, this group was less likely to report their injury, for fear of losing play time. There are many possibilities that could explain the apparent association between headband use and decreased risk of concussion. Until further medical studies are conducted, no definitive conclusions regarding the use of soccer headbands to reduce the risk of concussion can be reached.

PLAYING SURFACE

Some investigators have suggested that the type of playing surface may affect the rates of concussion or the severity of concussions. In a study published in 2002 in the *Journal of Trauma*, Rosanne Naunheim investigated the peak acceleration after impact on three different playing surfaces: natural grass, the indoor artificial turf of a practice field, and the indoor artificial turf in a domed stadium. Her results showed that peak acceleration was greatest with the indoor artificial turf of the domed stadium at 262 Gs, compared to 246 Gs for natural grass and 184 Gs for artificial turf on the indoor practice field. These results suggest that the type of surface on which a game is played may affect the risk of sustaining a concussion after a fall to the ground.

In 2000, a study published by athletic trainer Kevin Guskiewicz examined the effect that playing surface had on immediate signs and symptoms of concussion. The results suggested that those athletes who sustained their concussions on artificial turf were more likely to lose consciousness than those athletes playing on natural grass.

The data published thus far regarding playing surface and risk of concussion are preliminary. Furthermore, the type of surface on which athletes play is determined by many factors other than the risk of concussion. Expense, upkeep, space, location, and weather patterns, all factor into a program's decision about which playing surface to use. Still, further research could clarify the effects of playing surface on concussion risk. Once clarified, programs could consider concussion risk as one of the factors used to help determine which playing surface they will employ.

Although some may find it discouraging, readers of this text can deduce an obvious explanation for the limitation in protective equipment in reducing concussion risk. For a moment, let us consider the way a shin guard works in soccer. When a soccer player without a shin guard is kicked by an opponent in the shin, a tremendous amount of force is delivered to the point on the shin struck by the toe box of his opponent's shoe. This blow to the shin causes significant pain, bruising, and occasionally fracture of the underlying shin bone.

When the shin is covered by a shin guard, the amount of force delivered to the shin is the same. But rather than being delivered to one point on the shin, the force is now distributed over a larger surface area, specifically, the size of the shin guard. Thus, the force is absorbed by a larger area of the shin. This decreases pain, bruising, and overall injury.

Helmets operate in a similar way. Nearly the same amount of force strikes the player's head. But rather than the force being focused at the point of impact, it is distributed over the larger surface area of the helmet. We have already learned that concussion results from a rapid, rotational acceleration of the brain, or spinning, as a result of an impact. Helmets distribute the force of an impact over a wider surface area. But they do little to reduce the overall force. Therefore, they do little to reduce the resulting acceleration. Since it is the acceleration of the brain that causes the concussion, helmets can do little to reduce the risk of concussion. Newer technologies are attempts to reduce the acceleration after impact. Whether they will be effective at reducing the risk of concussions in sports remains to be seen.

It is true that foam used to line the inside of sport helmets does reduce the force to a small degree by the time it reaches the player's head. This reduction, however, is small. It appears that such a small reduction in force does not significantly reduce the incidence of concussion in these sports.

In summary, there is currently no reliable medical evidence showing that personal protective equipment reduces an athlete's risk of sustaining a sport-related concussion. Both scientific and medical investigations are underway to try and develop such personal protective devices. Hopefully, some effective equipment will be developed over the next decade or two. While they may not be proven to reduce the risk of concussion, however, helmets, mouth guards, and other personal protective devices are extremely effective at reducing the risk of catastrophic brain injuries, skull and facial bone fractures, dental injury, scalp lacerations, as well as other injuries. Therefore, all athletes participating in sports should wear all appropriate, protective equipment recommended by the governing administrative bodies. In addition, all such personal protective equipment should be new, in proper working condition, and fitted appropriately.

Suggested Readings

Biasca, N., S. Wirth, and Y. Tegner. The avoidability of head and neck injuries in ice hockey: An historical review. *Br J Sports Med*, 2002, 36(6): 410–427.

Blignaut, J. B., I. L. Carstens, and C. J. Lombard, Injuries sustained in rugby by wearers and non-wearers of mouthguards. *Br J Sports Med*, 1987, 21(2): 5–7.

Concussions and the marketing of sports equipment. Hearing before the Committee on Commerce, Science, and Transportation United States Senate, One Hundred Twelfth Congress, First Session, October 19, 2011. https://www.gpo.gov/fdsys/pkg/chrg-112shrg73514/pdf/chrg-112shrg73514.pdf.

McIntosh, A. S., and P. McCrory. Impact energy attenuation performance of football headgear. *Br J Sports Med,* 2000, 34(5): 337–341.

Mihalik, J. P., et al. Effectiveness of mouthguards in reducing neurocognitive deficits following sports-related cerebral concussion. *Dent Traumatol,* 2007, 23(1): 14–20.

Naunheim, R., et al. Does the use of artificial turf contribute to head injuries? *J Trauma,* 2002, 53(4): 691–694.

Theye, F., and K. A. Mueller. "Heads up": Concussions in high school sports. *Clin Med Res,* 2004, 2(3): 165–171.

5

NEW MEDICAL INFORMATION: WHY CONCUSSION IS TAKEN SO SERIOUSLY NOW

Ted Johnson played linebacker for the New England Patriots. He was a hard-hitting, energetic, dynamic player, and a fan favorite. On August 10, 2002, during an exhibition game against the New York Giants, he sustained one of the many concussions that he suffered during his career. In a 2007 interview with *Boston Globe* reporter Jackie MacMullan, Johnson described the hit he delivered to Giant's running back, Sean Bennett, as "a terrific collision." It was a high-energy impact which resulted in Johnson being confused and blacking out.

Before the season had even started, Ted Johnson was concussed.

He was pulled from the game after discussing his injury with Patriots medical staff. But several days later, despite suffering from persistent symptoms, he was pressured to return. He marks this as the start of his precipitous decline.

The remainder of his story is well known, having been described in several news articles, on several television shows, and featured on HBO's *Real Sports with Bryant Gumbel*. He reports suffering from crippling depression and apathy, often going days on end without shaving, showering, brushing his teeth, or leaving his apartment. He is, at times, unable to keep appointments. He and his physician, Dr. Robert Cantu, a world famous neurosurgeon and an expert in the management of concussive brain injuries, attribute Johnson's symptoms to the multiple concussions he sustained while playing football. And his symptoms are extensive, including, depression, fatigue, difficulty concentrating, poor memory, and ringing in the ears, among others. While he told the *Boston Globe* he has only been diagnosed officially with three or four concussions, Johnson estimates he has suffered more than 30, adding, "I have been dinged so many times I've lost count."

This chapter will review the reasons why concussive brain injuries, and sport-related concussions in particular, are taken more seriously nowadays than they were years ago. Both medical and scientific studies will be reviewed.

There are four main reasons why concussion is taken much more seriously nowadays then it was 25 years ago.

1. Athletes who sustain one concussion are at a higher risk for getting another than athletes who have never had a concussion.
2. The effects of concussions are, to some extent, cumulative, meaning the more concussions athletes have, the worse their brain function becomes after each injury, and the longer it takes for them to recover from each concussion.
3. Some athletes who sustain concussions will develop problems later in life such as dementia, confusion, depression, and other problems. Some athletes with these problems have been diagnosed at autopsy with an entity now known as "chronic traumatic encephalopathy" (CTE).
4. Athletes, particularly young male athletes, who return to sport before complete recovery from a concussion, are at risk for life-threatening swelling of the brain known as "second impact syndrome."

INCREASED RISK

Several studies have shown that athletes who have sustained one concussion are at increased risk for sustaining more. In 1977, a woman named Susan Gerberich investigated the number of concussions that occurred during high school football in Minnesota. She asked athletes to complete a questionnaire assessing details about their recent football season. She received responses from 3,063 players, representing 81 percent of those who received the questionnaire. Overall, approximately 19 percent of football players sustained a concussion during the 1977 fall football season. From her results, she noticed that the risk of being knocked unconscious was four times higher for those athletes who had been knocked unconscious before than for athletes who had never lost consciousness.

During the 1970s, there was still significant debate about how "concussion" should be defined. However, physicians on both sides of the debate agreed that an athlete who lost consciousness had sustained a concussion. Therefore, in order to avoid debate, it was often useful to separate out concussions that involved a loss of consciousness from those that did not involve a loss of consciousness. Certainly, these findings drew some much needed attention to the issue of concussive brain injury in American football. An athlete who had been knocked unconscious previously in his lifetime was four times more likely to be knocked unconscious during a given football season than an athlete who had never lost consciousness. This finding suggested that, perhaps, athletes who had sustained a concussion previously were more likely to sustain an additional concussion.

During the late 1990s, a man named Mark Schulz collected data on nearly 16,000 athletes in North Carolina high schools and revealed a similar finding: those athletes who had sustained concussions in the past were twice as likely to sustain a concussion during the study period than those athletes who had never had a concussion. Several differences in the study by Schulz are worth noting. First of all, Schulz looked at all concussions, not only those that involved a loss of consciousness. Although some debate still existed in the late 1990s, it was more generally accepted that concussions occurred even when an athlete did not lose consciousness. Furthermore, Schulz looked not only at American football, but other sports as well, including those played by female athletes. This drew some much needed attention to the risk of concussive brain injury in sports other than American football.

Similar results have been seen in studies of collegiate athletes. Kevin Guskiewicz, a scientist and athletic trainer from the University of North Carolina, followed nearly 3,000 college football players over the course of three seasons. His results showed that college football players with previous concussions were three times more likely to sustain a concussion than their teammates who had no previous concussions.

As these and other medical investigations revealed similar findings, the medical community realized that an athlete who has sustained a concussion at some point during his or her lifetime is at increased risk for sustaining sport-related concussions in the future when compared to athletes who have never had a concussion. The reasons for this increased risk are unknown. There are several possibilities.

A. It could be that some athletes are born with some predisposition or vulnerability to concussive brain injury. Perhaps the substance of their brain, the shape of their skull, or other physical characteristics make them more likely to sustain a concussion. When these athletes are included in medical studies, they are more likely to have sustained a concussion prior to the start of the medical study, since they are predisposed. Similarly, they are more likely to sustain a concussion during the medical study, simply because they are predisposed to concussive injury. Note, this increased risk has nothing to do with their prior injury. They are simply born predisposed to sustaining concussive brain injury. They have always been at higher risk.

B. It could be that it is simply a matter of playing time. Perhaps, athletes who receive more play-time sustain more concussions because they are more often at risk. The athlete on the ice playing hockey, or on the field playing football, is more likely to sustain an injury than the athlete on the bench, riding the pine. Thus, athletes who receive more play time are more likely to an injured prior to the start of the study and more likely to get injured over the course of the study.

C. It could be a matter of playing style. Perhaps athletes who sustain more concussions are too aggressive, constantly flinging themselves recklessly into risky situations. Perhaps they often lead with their heads, placing themselves at greater risk of concussion. Or, maybe they are not aggressive enough. Maybe they are somewhat timid. As a result, a more aggressive player lines them up and delivers a well-timed, coordinated blow that not only renders them incapable of performing their competitive duties, but also results in a concussion.

D. It may be a matter of body mass. Studies done in pee-wee and bantam ice hockey leagues have shown that athletes who are smaller in size are at increased risk for concussion compared to their larger counterparts. Perhaps smaller athletes sustain more concussions than larger athletes simply because they sustain more blows delivered by larger athletes capable of producing larger forces.

E. Finally, it could be that once athletes sustain a concussion, something changes in the brain that predisposes them to future concussions. This final possibility results in a great deal of concern for those of us engaged in athletics, sports medicine, and the management of concussive brain injury.

Currently, those of us in the medical field do not known which of these possibilities is true. It could be that all of these explanations are true, each accounting for some proportion of repeat concussions sustained by athletes. No matter the reason, athletes who have sustained one or more concussions are at increased risk for additional concussions. As a result, they should be managed closely, with all available technologies.

CUMULATIVE EFFECTS

The effects of concussion are cumulative. There is some lasting effect on the brain after a concussion that persists, even after the athlete feels better. Athletes who sustain multiple concussions will have more significant symptoms, a more impressive decrease in their overall brain function, and will often take longer to recover than athletes who sustain only one concussion. Several medical studies have led to this conclusion.

A neuropsychologist is a clinician and scientist who has a doctoral degree in measuring brain function. In the 1970s, a neuropsychologist named Dorothy Gronwall measured the brain function of patients referred to her clinic after having sustained a concussion. She separated these patients into groups. One group consisted of patients who had sustained two concussions during their lifetime. The other group consisted of patients who had sustained only one concussion during their lifetime. She then measured the brain functions of the patients, and compared their performance. She found that those patients who were referred to her office after sustaining their second lifetime concussion had worse brain function than those who had sustained only one concussion. Furthermore, it took longer for the brain function of those who had sustained two lifetime concussions to return to normal than it did for patients who had sustained only one lifetime concussion. She concluded that the effects of concussion, therefore, are cumulative. These results suggested that there are some lasting effects on the brain after a concussion that do not resolve. At the very minimum, these effects make subsequent injuries more significant and more difficult to recover from.

Studies in athletes have shown similar findings. In the same study by Kevin Guskiewicz noted previously, athletes took longer to recover from a concussion if they had sustained a concussion previously. Only 15 percent of players with one prior concussion had symptoms that lasted longer than a week. But for players who had three or more prior concussions, 30 percent had symptoms lasting longer than a week.

Even the events that occur at the time of injury may be different for athletes who have sustained multiple concussions when compared to those who have sustained only one concussion. In a study performed by Micky Collins, a neuropsychologist at the University of Pittsburgh Medical Center, athletes who sustained a concussion were more likely to be knocked unconscious, to suffer confusion, and to suffer amnesia, if they had sustained prior concussions.

These findings are true whether or not the prior concussions have been formally diagnosed by medical personnel. In a joint study of athletes cared for at Boston Children's Hospital and the University of Pittsburgh Medical Center, nearly one third of athletes who presented for care of a sport-related concussion had sustained a previous concussion that went undiagnosed. Athletes who sustained concussions that went undiagnosed were at risk for more severe symptoms and loss of consciousness at the time of their most recent concussions compared to those athletes who are presenting with their first ever concussion.

It should be obvious to most readers that athletes are at constant risk for sustaining a concussion, particularly those involved in contact or collision sports. Therefore, athletes who sustain multiple concussions often sustain them within a relatively short time period. In fact, in the study by Kevin Guskiewicz, 90 percent of athletes who sustained repeat concussions during the same season suffered their repeat injuries within 10 days of one another. Furthermore, at the time these studies were conducted, many athletes were returned to sports before they were fully recovered from their concussions. This has led some to speculate that there is not, in fact, a cumulative effect of multiple concussive brain injuries when an athlete has proper time to recover in between each concussion. If an athlete has proper time to recover from one concussion before sustaining another concussion, some argue, there would be no measurable effects from the previous injury. The athlete would recover just as quickly as if he or she had only sustained only one concussion. The deficits in brain function would be no different than if the athlete had only sustained one concussion. This leaves open the possibility that if athletes fully recover in between their concussions, they might not develop these cumulative effects. It is possible that recovering fully between injuries might minimize any potential, cumulative effects of injury. This hopeful possibility is one of the reasons why athletic trainers, doctors, and neuropsychologists recommend avoiding contact or collision sports until an athlete is completely recovered from a concussion.

It is interesting to note, however, that Dorothy Gronwall was not only studying athletes. Rather, she was studying all patients referred to her clinic with a concussion. Outside of sports, concussion is a relatively rare injury. It is uncommon for people who are not engaged in athletics to sustain a concussion. Certainly, having more than one concussion over the course of a lifetime is uncommon for non-athletes. Therefore the length of time in between injuries tends to be greater for patients not playing sports than it is for patients playing sports. In Gronwall's study, the time in between concussions for those patients who had sustained two concussions ranged from five months to eight years. The average length of time in between the two concussions was 4.5 years. Therefore, statistically, it is likely that the majority of her patients, if not all of her patients, had recovered completely from the first injury at the time they sustained their second. Despite this, she was able to detect worse brain function and longer recovery times for those who sustained their second concussion. This suggests that there is, in fact, some cumulative, permanent effect on the brain after a concussion regardless of the amount of time an athlete or patient has to recover in between injuries. It should be noted that this effect is small, particularly for concussions sustained during sports. In fact, it is often difficult to detect any effect at all until athletes sustain additional concussions at which point it is noted that the symptoms seem to be more intense and last for a longer period of time, on average, than athletes who are sustaining their first lifetime concussion. It is also important to note that these studies are conducted on multiple players. For an individual athlete, the second concussion may cause less severe symptoms and may be associated with a shorter recovery than the first. When taken collectively, however, it is clear that athletes who have sustained prior concussions will experience more severe symptoms and longer recovery times, on average, than athletes who have sustained their first.

While further research needs to be conducted into the potential effect of complete recovery in between injuries, most clinicians agree that an athlete who completely recovers in between concussions is better off than the athlete who sustains an additional concussion before completely recovering from a prior concussion. Animal models of repeated concussion have shown that increasing the interval between injuries decreases the long-term effects on brain function, particularly learning and memory. There is also clinical evidence that symptom severity and duration of symptoms are exacerbated by concussions that occurred during the previous year, but that if more than a year has elapsed, clean the prior concussion and injury under study, the effect is minimal. In addition, completely recovering from a concussion prior to sustaining an additional concussion decreases, if not completely eliminates, the risk of second impact syndrome, a catastrophic injury often leading to death, coma, or permanent loss of brain function, which will be discussed later in this chapter.

LONG-TERM EFFECTS

Many readers will remember classmates from their youth who spoke a little more slowly than others, seemed a little "spacey" or "out of it." When these students played sports like football or boxing, people used to say things like "that guy took too many hits to the head," or "that guy got his bell rung one time too many." The term "punch drunk" was fairly common. This may be a case, as often happens, where common sense and intuition precede medical knowledge. Although these remarks were often made jokingly, there was some understanding, some belief, that multiple concussions could result in problems with brain function, slowed thinking, slowed speaking, poor concentration, etc. Medical scientific studies are starting to confirm these previous suspicions.

Although the attention of the medical community has only recently been drawn to the long-term effects of concussive brain injury, one of the first medical articles to note the potential long-term effects of multiple blows to the head was published in 1928, in the *Journal of the American Medical Association*. In his article entitled "Punch Drunk," a physician named Harrison Martland detailed the physical characteristics of certain boxers described by fans as being "cuckoo, goofy, . . . slug nutty." The boxers Martland described developed an abnormal way of walking, where the men would drag a leg slightly behind them. Some would progress to develop more general slowing of all of their movements. Martland noticed these boxers had slowed speech, shaking of their hands, involuntary nodding of their heads. Some were unable to show expressions on their faces which became somewhat mask-like in their appearance. He reported that these men were often mistaken for being drunk. One such boxer was even excluded from a fight because he was suspected of being drunk at the time, when, in actuality, he was sober. Some of these pugilists became worse with time, losing the ability to think properly, to function in the world, to hold a job. Some were ultimately hospitalized in an asylum.

Martland observed that this disease was seen mostly in boxers who were known for their ability to take a punch. "Punch drunk" syndrome was uncommon in speedy, skilled, elusive fighters whose goal was to outbox their opponents by scoring more points by landing more punches. Given their skill and agility, these types of boxers sustained relatively few square punches to the head. Rather, the illness Martland described was seen in boxers of the "slugging type," men who endured considerable blows to the head but managed to stay on their feet, engaged in the fight, seeking to land one giant knockout blow in order to win.

Those of you unfamiliar with boxing, but who have seen the movies Rocky or Rocky 2, can still appreciate these two separate styles of boxing. Apollo Creed would be the skilled, agile, elusive fighter. His ultimate goal is to outbox Rocky Balboa. Creed is constantly bobbing and weaving, dodging the slow yet forceful punches of Balboa. Creed rarely sustains a square punch to the head. Rocky Balboa, on the other hand, is a boxer of the "slugging type." He is not as fast, skilled, or agile as Creed. He cannot possibly hope to out-box Apollo Creed. But given his enormous strength and power, he seeks to win the bout by delivering one, powerful, fatal knockout blow that knocks Creed unconscious for 10 seconds. Balboa endures considerable punishment, sustaining multiple blows to the head and body, yet remains on his feet in the hopes of delivering that one, mighty, winning blow. Balboa can take a punch. It is in this type of fighter, "the slugger," represented by Balboa, that Martland described the entity he called "punch drunk."

The characteristics of "punch drunk" as described by Martland are similar to those described more recently in former professional football players ultimately diagnosed with CTE. This entity will be discussed further in Chapter 12.

Full-blown "punch drunk" syndrome or CTE, however, may not be the only effect of multiple blows to the head, or multiple concussions. A well-known study by athletic trainer, Kevin Guskiewicz, examined the proportion of retired American football players with impaired brain function later in life. He found that players who had sustained multiple concussions were three times more likely to report problems with memory than those who did not sustain concussions. Furthermore, his results showed that the rates of brain dysfunction in retired football players who sustained three or more concussions during their career were five times higher than retired football players who did not sustain a concussion during their career. Those retired football players who had developed Alzheimer's disease did so at a younger age than the general American male population. It should be noted that these players played football during an era when concussions were diagnosed and managed much differently than they are today. It is possible, even likely, that today's standards for recognizing, diagnosing, and treating concussion likely reduce the potential for cumulative effects. In addition, while these findings are concerning for long-term effects of concussions, there have also been studies that did not detect any long-term effects from sport-related concussions. As a result, there is ongoing controversy about whether concussions result in any long-term problems.

Most athletes who sustain sport-related concussions make full and complete recoveries, regaining all of their previous brain function. It is possible, however, that some athletes, as a result of multiple concussive brain injuries, lose some brain function that they never recover. The differences between these two groups of athletes are unclear at this time. There are several possibilities:

1. Those who have lost some brain function may have sustained many more concussions than those who have retained their brain function.
2. Those who have lost brain function may have sustained injuries that involved greater forces than those who have retained their cognitive function.
3. Some people may be more vulnerable to the effects of concussion, such that they have a more difficult time recovering their brain function after a concussion, or after multiple concussions. This vulnerability may be due to their genetics, the shape of their brain, the shape of their skull, or other factors.
4. Those who have lost some brain function may have sustained repeated injuries without recovering fully in between each of them, while those who retain their brain function recovered fully in between their concussions.
5. There may be a certain age at which sustaining concussions results in a loss of brain function that is not recoverable, while athletes at different ages at the time of their concussions are able to fully recover.

One of the jobs of physicians, scientists, neuropsychologists, athletic trainers and others involved in the care of athletes is to discover the reasons why certain athletes lose some of the capabilities of their brain as a result of sustaining concussions, while other do not. Such insights might lead to prevention and treatment strategies.

SECOND IMPACT SYNDROME

Although rare, second impact syndrome is tragic.

In 1984, two physicians named Saunders and Harbaugh described the tragic case of a man who died after sustaining a head injury. He was a 19 year old college student and football player. He had been in a fistfight during which he received a blow to the head that knocked him unconscious. The day after the fistfight, he was taken to the school infirmary where he had headaches and nausea. He was removed from football. Three days later he reported feeling better but still had a mild headache. He returned to football. During a play in which no one recalls any significant trauma to the head, or other major blow to the body, the patient became ill. He walked off the field and collapsed. He was taken to an emergency department, where he was noted to be unconscious. A breathing tube was inserted so that doctors could help maintain his breathing. He had a picture of his brain called computed tomography (CT) or "cat scan." It showed significant swelling of the brain and a small amount of blood. He died several days later, despite medical and surgical treatments. Saunders and Harbaugh hypothesized that because this young man had not fully recovered from his prior concussion that he had sustained during the fistfight, he was more susceptible to the catastrophic swelling of the brain that resulted from a blow so minor that none of his teammates could recall it.

Since that time, there have been multiple similar cases described in the medical literature. This occurrence has become known as second impact syndrome.

An athlete who is recovering from a concussion, but is not yet fully recovered, is at risk for second impact syndrome. When athletes return to play before they are fully recovered from a concussion, a second blow to the head, even a mild one, or even a blow to the body that results in a rapid movement of the head, can cause massive swelling in the brain. Since the brain is contained in the rigid bone of the skull, this swelling causes compression of the brain. In severe cases, the brain is squeezed through small holes within the skull. This squeezing of the brain through these small holes is known as "herniation." Herniation can lead to decreased blood flow to the brain, and ultimately to the athlete's death.

Every year during football season, there is an article in the newspaper about an athlete who returned to football before he had recovered completely from a concussion. Often, the athlete told his doctor, athletic trainer and coach that he was better but confided to friends and teammates that he still had some lingering symptoms, such as headaches or nausea. And, although no one remembers any major blows to the head or collisions, the athlete develops massive brain swelling and dies.

Although second impact syndrome is rare, it has a devastating effect on those involved. Those who do survive second impact syndrome are neurologically devastated. They often spend many weeks to months in a coma. Many times they have a hole cut in their neck through which a permanent breathing tube is inserted. They are hooked up to a machine to help them breathe. They receive all of their nutrition intravenously as they are not awake enough or alert enough to eat or drink. The athletic trainer, team physician, primary care physician, and other medical personnel are left wondering about their relationship with the athlete. Oftentimes, they are confused as to why the athlete would not tell them about his symptoms. They question whether there were other steps they could have taken in order to prevent the injury. They start to fear that other athletes on the team are perhaps downplaying their symptoms in order to return to play and are therefore at risk for second impact syndrome. They are often reluctant to allow future athletes to return after sustaining a sport-related concussion. The coaching staff suffers many of the same emotions. They too are left wondering whether their coaching had something to do with the athlete downplaying his symptoms. They wonder whether there was anything they could have done to prevent the injury. They worry about the remainder of athletes under their supervision. Second impact syndrome is perhaps hardest on the teammates of the injured player. While some of them were often aware that the athlete was still experiencing symptoms from his concussion, most were unaware that returning to play prior to complete recovery from a concussion could lead to such a devastating outcome. They often feel a sense of guilt about not informing the athletic trainer, parents, or coaching staff that the athlete was still experiencing symptoms. They are devastated by the loss of their friend. They are haunted by thoughts that perhaps they could have prevented the injury. They fear for their own safety on the playing field.

Avoiding second impact syndrome is one of the main reasons why medical professionals do not return athletes to sports until their symptoms have completely resolved.

Something else is worth noting about the case described by Saunders and Harbaugh. The athlete sustained his concussion in a fistfight, outside of organized athletic activity. While those of us in sports medicine concentrate on concussions that occur during sports, athletes can also sustain concussions outside of organized, supervised athletics. Given the lack of parental or medical supervision during these instances, diagnosing these concussions is even more difficult, especially without the help of the athlete. These circumstances should not be overlooked. Furthermore, when an athlete reports a concussion that was sustained outside of athletics, those of us involved in sports medicine are often still the best equipped to manage the injury.

Thus far, second impact syndrome has only been described in boys and young men. Perhaps there is something different about the male brain, or more specifically the young male brain, which predisposes it to second impact syndrome. It could be that male athletes are susceptible to this injury, whereas female athletes are not. I suspect, however, that girls, women, and older men are as equally susceptible to second impact syndrome. But since the majority of athletes playing contact and collision sports are young men and boys, and since second impact syndrome is rare, it is statistically more likely to occur in young male athletes. But the overall numbers of female athletes participating in contact and collision sports is increasing every year. It is possible that a case of second impact syndrome will occur in a female athlete in the future.

In summary, those who sustain one concussion are at increased risk of future concussions than those who have never suffered a concussion. The effects of multiple concussions are likely cumulative. For some athletes, there are long-term effects from sustaining multiple concussions. Second impact syndrome is a devastating injury, often resulting in death, sustained by athletes who have not yet recovered from a concussion when they receive a second impact, often minor, that leads to a rapid acceleration of the head. It is characterized by massive swelling of the brain that can cause the brain to be squeezed through small holes within the skull. Second impact syndrome often leads to death. Those who survive are neurologically devastated. It has thus far only been reported in boys and young men. But this may simply be due to the large number of boys and young men at risk for it. Cases in women or older men may be seen in the future.

Suggested Readings

Collins, M. W., et al. Relationship between concussion and neuropsychological performance in college football players. *JAMA*, 1999, 282(10): 964–970.

Eisenberg, M., J. Andrea, W. P. Meehan, III, and R. Mannix. Time interval between concussions and symptom duration. *Pediatrics*, 2013, 132(1): 8–17.

Gerberich, S. G., et al. Concussion incidences and severity in secondary school varsity football players. *Am J Public Health*, 1983, 73(12): 1370–1375.

Guskiewicz, K. M., et al. Cumulative effects associated with recurrent concussion in collegiate football players: The NCAA Concussion Study. *JAMA*, 2003, 290(19): 2549–2455.

Martland, H. Punch drunk. *JAMA*, 1928, 91(15): 1103–1107.

Meehan, W. P., III, R. C. Mannix, M. J. O'Brien, and M. W. Collins. The prevalence of undiagnosed concussions in athletes. *Clin J Sport Med*, 2013, 23(5): 339–342.

Meehan, W. P., III, J. Zhang, R. Mannix, and M. J. Whalen. Increasing recovery time between injuries improves cognitive outcome after repeat mild concussions in mice. *Neurosurgery*, 2012, 71(4): 885–892.

Saunders, R. L., and R. E. Harbaugh. The second impact in catastrophic contact-sports head trauma. *JAMA*, 1984, 252(4): 538–539.

6

"NEUROPSYCHOLOGICAL" OR "NEUROCOGNITIVE" TESTING: WHAT IT IS AND WHICH ATHLETES SHOULD HAVE IT

On September 26, 2009, the Florida Gators were beating the Kentucky Wildcats by a score of 31 to 7. It was the third quarter. The Gators star quarterback, Tim Tebow, called for the snap. He was looking to his right, when, from his blind side, he was drilled by Kentucky's number 94, Tyler Wyndham, who charged, unblocked, from the line of scrimmage. Wyndham's helmet struck Tebow's facemask, rocketing his head backward. As he was pinned to the ground, his head bounced forward off of the leg of his teammate, Marcus Gilbert. As he lay on the field, he flinched once or twice, but was mostly motionless. It was several minutes before Tebow could be removed from the field. On the sidelines, he started to vomit. He was taken to a nearby hospital where he had a CT of the brain, which was negative for bleeding. He was admitted overnight.

Tim Tebow was concussed.

The media coverage that followed Tebow's concussion was uncommon. Perhaps because of Tebow's stature and fame, his concussion received more media coverage than most. There was some good that came out of the coverage. Many younger athletes saw that Tebow was taken out of the game. Many sports fans unfamiliar with concussion management read about Tebow's "baseline" test and how he would retake it later, when doctors felt he was improving, to help assess when he was recovered. For many, this was the first they had ever heard of neuropsychological testing.

The terms neuropsychological testing and neurocognitive testing are often used interchangeably. When discussed in the context of athletes sustaining sport-related concussions, these terms mostly refer to computerized neurocognitive testing.

Neuropsychology is a long-standing profession dating back to the earliest times of research in brain function. It is a subspecialty of psychology that deals with the function of the brain and how it relates to behavior. Neuropsychologists are clinician-scientists who assess brain functioning. They use standard tests to determine patients' cognitive, social, emotional, and behavioral functioning. They measure patients' reaction time and the speed with which patients solve problems. They assess patients' decisions, decision-making abilities, and the strategies patients use to make decisions. The data obtained during these observations and tests allow neuropsychologists to understand how a patient's brain is working. These measurements of brain function can be used to help determine appropriate treatments and interventions, clarify diagnoses, and assess relative strengths and weaknesses in many conditions such as attention deficit hyperactivity disorder, learning disabilities, autism, Alzheimer's disease, and epilepsy (recurrent seizures). They can be used to assess brain function after injuries such as stroke, drowning, and traumatic brain injuries. In the setting of sports, they are most often used to measure brain function before and after a sport-related concussion.

In the 1980s, a group of neuropsychologists suggested measuring brain function in athletes who played American football. Given the large number of athletes playing American football, and the relatively high occurrence of concussions in American football, it seemed logical. Since that time, there have been numerous medical studies investigating the use of neuropsychological testing in assessing sport-related concussions.

In 1999, a landmark study was published in the *Journal of the American Medical Association* (*JAMA*). In this study, a neuropsychologist named Micky Collins, and his colleagues at the University of Pittsburgh Medical Center measured the brain function of 393 college football players prior to the start of a football season. Those athletes who sustained a concussion during the season were retested after their injuries. The results were remarkable.

Prior to the start of the season, those athletes who had sustained a concussion at some point during their life, performed worse on neuropsychological tests then those athletes who had never sustained a concussion. This has led some to suggest that the effects of concussion are permanent and do not resolve with time. But this cannot be concluded from these data. It is possible that the lower brain functioning measured by the tests was present before the injuries and perhaps predisposed these athletes to sustaining a concussion rather than resulted from their previous concussions. Indeed, it is not hard to imagine that athletes with slower reaction times might be at increased risk for a sport-related concussion. Similarly, however, we can just as easily imagine that multiple concussions themselves led to permanently slower reaction times. Other studies, discussed later in this book, have been performed to address this question. The study by Dr. Collins and his colleagues showed convincingly, however, that concussion results in abnormal brain function after injury. This was not commonly accepted at the time of this publication.

This study required an enormous amount of work. The neuropsychological tests took 30 minutes or more to perform for each athlete. They tested nearly 400 football players. So, while the results were revealing, it did not seem like a practical way to assess or monitor sport-related concussions among the very large population of athletes who are at risk for sustaining sport-related concussions. Many college football teams have 70–100 players. Testing each of them before the start of the season would require one or more trained neuropsychologists to spend 35–50 hours examining the athletes. A written report would have to be generated for each athlete. After each concussion, the tests would have to be repeated, often multiple times, while monitoring recovery. The team would have to pay for each test. Routinely allotting this amount of time in an already packed athletic training schedule would be difficult. While professional and some major college athletic programs might have the funding for such an endeavor, few, if any, high schools would. Furthermore, concussion occurs in other sports besides American football. The thought of performing these traditional neuropsychological assessments on every at-risk athlete at the beginning of each season, and again, often multiple times, after each concussive injury, seemed daunting. Indeed, it was unlikely to happen on a large scale.

The constraints of traditional neuropsychological testing led to the invention of computerized neurocognitive tests. These tests use a computer to measure brain function in place of some of the previous versions of traditional neuropsychological tests. Computerized versions have several advantages over the traditional testing paradigms. They allow for multiple preseason or "baseline" tests to be performed simultaneously. If there are enough computers available, the entire team can be tested at once. Since they are limited in their scope, medical personnel such as team physicians and certified athletic trainers can be taught to administer and perform limited interpretations of the tests. Computerized tests are more affordable than traditional tests. And they are more precise in certain areas of testing. For example, the computerized tests can measure an athlete's reaction time to 1/1000th of a second, much more precisely than a person with a clock or stopwatch can measure.

While taking computerized neurocognitive tests, athletes are asked to complete several tasks. Often, they are given a series of words to remember. Periodically throughout the duration of the test, the athlete is asked to recall whether various words were a part of the original list. A similar list of designs or shapes is also presented, and athletes are asked periodically to recall whether various shapes were a part of the original list. There are tasks of memory and concentration, similar in many ways to the card game "concentration" that many readers will have played during their childhood, where athletes are asked to remember the location of various objects after they have been covered. There are tests dealing with numbers, letters, and various designs. Measurements are recorded of the number of tasks performed correctly, the number performed incorrectly, and the time it takes for athletes to complete each task. From these measurements, clinicians can obtain a quantitative measurement of the athlete's cognitive abilities. This is stored in the medical record.

Ideally, the athletes on teams engaging in sports with a significant risk of concussion will each undergo a baseline computerized neurocognitive test prior to the start of the season. This will be considered a measurement of their normal brain function, the functioning that their brain is capable of when it is not injured. Then, if an athlete sustains a concussion during the season, the test is repeated. This allows doctors, athletic trainers, and neuropsychologists to see how far the athlete's function has decreased. Furthermore, the test can be repeated to monitor recovery. Medical personnel can see how long it takes for the athlete to regain his or her preseason functioning.

While computerized neurocognitive tests are valuable in assessing and managing sport-related concussions, they should not be viewed as a replacement for traditional neuropsychological testing. In traditional testing, a trained neuropsychologist is able to detect aspects of brain functioning by observing how a patient approaches certain problems, handles difficulties, and processes information. During traditional testing, the neuropsychologists can interact with the patient to gain an understanding of how he or she is handling a given task. This direct observation and interaction is lost with computerized testing. In addition, these tests are currently used mostly for the detection, assessment and management of traumatic brain injury. Their potential role in other disease processes and other diagnoses is not yet clear. Finally, their interpretation is limited by the training and experience of the clinician using them. Physicians and athletic trainers can be taught to administer and interpret these tests to some extent. They can administer baseline tests and determine the validity of baseline tests. They can be taught to detect variations from baseline performance after injury and return to baseline performance during recovery from concussion. They can even be trained to detect some of the more common mistakes and misinterpretations of the directions by athletes, and learn how to correct for those mistakes by mathematically adjusting the patient's scores. There is, however, little doubt that a trained neuropsychologist who has significant training and experience using computerized neurocognitive testing will be able to glean more information from these tests. Such neuropsychologists are better equipped to interpret tests complicated by learning disabilities, attention deficit hyperactivity disorder, and other factors that affect computerized neurocognitive test scores. Ideally, all concussion action plans will include the services of a neuropsychologist with specific training in the administration and interpretation of computerized neurocognitive tests.

For those who know how to properly administer and interpret these tests, they are highly valuable. Multiple medical studies have shown that these studies can help diagnose sport-related concussions and monitor recovery. Perhaps their most valuable quality is their ability to detect decreased brain function even after athletes report being symptom-free. Medical studies suggest that up to 20 percent of athletes who feel recovered from their sport-related concussions and report that they are symptom-free still have measurable deficits in their brain function for several additional days.

Prior to the routine use of neuropsychological testing in athletes at risk for sport-related concussions, athletic trainers and physicians managed these patients according to their symptoms. When athletes sustained a concussion and told their team medical personnel about it, they were removed from play. These athletes would complain of headaches, nausea, poor concentration, and other symptoms of concussion. Once they informed the team's medical personnel their symptoms had resolved, they were cleared to start the return to sports protocol. This left players vulnerable to three potential issues. First, many athletes do not recognize their symptoms as indicative of a concussion. Second, as discussed earlier, many athletes, for various reasons, report being symptom-free despite remaining symptomatic. Third, medical personnel had no way of knowing which athletes had persistent brain dysfunction, even after they reported being symptom-free. Computerized neurocognitive testing can help resolve each of these issues.

A study from the same group of investigators at the University of Pittsburgh Medical Center used computerized neuropsychological testing to assess the brain function of athletes prior to the start of the season, in what is now known as a "baseline" test, and after a concussion occurred, in what is now known as a "post-injury" test. Their study revealed that nearly 19 percent of athletes who reported having no residual symptoms after a sport-related concussion still had abnormal neuropsychological test scores. These findings are significant. They suggest that athletes who report being symptom-free have not always recovered their full brain function. Incorporating computerized neurocognitive testing into a full concussion management program allows sports medicine clinicians to detect those athletes who, despite reporting full resolution of their symptoms, are still concussed.

A few points should be noted about neuropsychological testing in the assessment and management of sport-related concussion. First, it is only one of several tools clinicians use when managing an athlete who has sustained a concussion. The assessment of sport-related concussions should also include: a thorough medical history detailing how the injury occurred and the details of previous concussions; a thorough neurological physical examination; a thorough and honest symptom inventory; and a standardized balance assessment. Limiting the assessment to only neuropsychological assessment denies athletes the safest and best medical care.

Too often, I hear news reporters saying an athlete is "taking a concussion test" to see if he can return to his given sport. This is a misleading statement. Athletes who perform well on these neuropsychological tests, even those who reachieve their baseline scores, will often require further recovery time. An athlete who is still experiencing symptoms, for example, will require further recovery time. Athletes who still have poor balance when compared to their preseason balance will require further recovery time. Athletes who have been out of training for several weeks or months due to their injury will need to regain their former conditioning, strength, agility, speed, timing, and coordination before returning to their activity. Finally, athletes who have sustained multiple concussions had severe symptoms after their concussions, significant cognitive dysfunction after their concussions, or prolonged recovery times will often require further time out of contact, even after their cognitive function has returned to baseline.

There is some debate as to when post-injury tests should be performed. If the test is being used solely to decide whether an athlete should be returned to play, then there is little point in conducting the test before the athlete's symptoms have completely resolved and his or her balance has been restored to its baseline level. Those athletes who still have poor balance or still have concussion symptoms will not be returned to sports no matter how well they perform on their neuropsychological tests. Thus, some clinicians will only perform these assessments when an athlete's symptoms have resolved and balance has been recovered. Neuropsychological tests, however, may have other uses. For example, student athletes will have homework, quizzes, tests, term papers, and other academic assignments during their recovery. Thus, when deciding how much schoolwork they should undertake, and which academic accommodations should be put into place, computerized neuropsychological tests can be helpful. They may be performed prior to symptom resolution and balance recovery under these circumstances. In some cases, where schools are reluctant to put academic accommodations in place, these tests can serve as objective, quantitative evidence that the athletes are suffering from cognitive dysfunction. This will often help to convince schools of the need for accommodations during the recovery period. Since memory is often worse after a concussion and the amount of time it takes to process information is often increased after concussion, scholar athletes may sustain a decrease in their grades if academic accommodations are not put in place. In order to help athletes suffering from a sport-related concussion keep up as best as they can with their schoolwork without any negative impact on their academic performance, academic accommodations are often put in place. Such accommodations frequently consist of extra time allowed for tests, quizzes, and completion of homework assignments and the postponement of major tests accounting for substantial proportion of a class grade until the athlete recovers.

Nearly all athletes should have baseline neuropsychological testing performed prior to the start of the season. When we first started the Sports Concussion Clinic in the Division of Sports Medicine at Children's Hospital Boston, it never occurred to me the type of athletes we would be seeing. Certainly, I expected to see athletes playing football, ice hockey, rugby, lacrosse, soccer, basketball, and baseball. But I didn't fully realize how many patients I would see who sustained their injuries cycling, horseback riding, skiing, snowboarding, figure skating, and cheerleading. And it never occurred to me I would see athletes who sustained their concussions from swimming, dancing, rowing crew, and sailing. The more I practice medicine, the more I realize concussion occurs in all sports. Therefore, I would recommend any athlete to seek baseline computerized neurocognitive testing.

Obviously, some sports carry a higher risk of concussion than others. I would strongly recommend baseline computerized neurocognitive testing for all athletes engaged in collision and combat sports. Collision sports are those sports in which the delivery of blows to the body is a purposeful part of the sport. Common examples of collision sports are:

American football
Boy's/men's ice hockey
Boy's/men's lacrosse
Rugby union
Rugby league
Australian rules football

Combat sports are those in which athletes are engaged in a fight, albeit with specific rules and guidelines, supervised by a referee. Common examples of combat sports are:

Boxing
Mixed martial arts
Karate
Judo
Wrestling

Furthermore, I would strongly recommend baseline testing for contact sports. Contact sports can be divided into two categories. Those in which contact occurs accidentally, meaning it is not a part of the activity, and those in which contact occurs incidentally, meaning it is a known, accepted part of the game, but purposeful blows are not delivered. Common examples of sports in which contact is possible but is rare and accidental are:

Skiing/snowboarding
Horseback riding
Pole vaulting
Sailing
Skateboarding
Bicycling
Gymnastics
Cheerleading
Springboard diving

Common examples of contact sports in which contact is an incidental but expected and accepted part of the game are:

Soccer
Baseball/softball
Basketball
Water polo
Women's/girls' lacrosse
Women's/girls' ice hockey
Field hockey

In addition, I strongly recommend that all athletes who have sustained *one* concussion at some point during their lifetime undergo baseline computerized neurocognitive testing after they have recovered and before they return to sports of any kind. As already discussed in this book, athletes who have sustained one concussion are at increased risk for another. Therefore, if possible, any athlete who has suffered one concussion should undergo computerized neurocognitive baseline assessment after he or she has recovered, before being cleared for participation in further sports activity. It would be unfortunate if these high-risk individuals were not managed with the best possible available means.

In summary, neuropsychological testing is used to assess an athlete's brain function both before and after injury. It is one of several tools used to diagnose a concussion, monitor recovery from a concussion, and safely return an athlete to play after a sport-related concussion. Computerized neurocognitive tests are accurate, convenient, and represent a huge advancement in the management of sport-related concussions. They enable sports medicine clinicians to detect an additional 20 percent of persistent concussions that may have been otherwise miscategorized as recovered. They are one of several tools used to assess and monitor recovery after a sport-related concussion. Most, if not all, athletes should undergo baseline neuropsychological testing. Athletes in high-risk sports and athletes who have sustained previous sport-related concussions should strongly consider having baseline neuropsychological testing performed.

SUGGESTED READINGS

Alves, W. M., R. W. Rimel, and W. E. Nelson. University of Virginia prospective study of football-induced minor head injury: Status report. *Clin Sports Med*, 1987, 6(1): 211–218.

Collins, M. W., et al. Relationship between concussion and neuropsychological performance in college football players. *JAMA*, 1999, 282(10): 964–970.

Echemendia, R. J. *Sports Neuropsychology: Assessment and Management of Traumatic Brain Injury*. New York: The Guilford Press, 2006.

Erlanger, D., et al. Development and validation of a web-based neuropsychological test protocol for sports-related return-to-play decision-making. *Arch Clin Neuropsychol*, 2003, 18(3): 293–316.

Erlanger, D. M., et al. Neuropsychology of sports-related head injury: Dementia pugilistica to post concussion syndrome. *Clin Neuropsychol*, 1999, 13(2): 193–209.

Meehan, W. P., III, P. d'Hemecourt, C. L. Collins, A. M. Taylor, and R. D. Comstock. Computerized neurocognitive testing for the management of sport-related concussions. *Pediatrics*, 2012, 129(1): 38–44.

Schatz, P. Long-term test-retest reliability of baseline cognitive assessments using ImPACT. *Am J Sports Med*, 38(1): 47–53.

Zohar, O., et al. Closed-head minimal traumatic brain injury produces long-term cognitive deficits in mice. *Neuroscience*, 2003, 118(4): 949–955.

7

THE ACUTE ASSESSMENT AND MANAGEMENT OF SPORT-RELATED CONCUSSION: WHAT HAPPENS WHEN AN ATHLETE SUSTAINS A CONCUSSION

Mixed martial arts fighters B. J. Penn and Caol Uno were nearly identical in weight at 154 pounds versus 153 pounds, respectively. Penn was approximately two inches taller. At the time, Uno had more experience. No one expected that the fight between them would last only 10 seconds.

In an exciting, energy-filled start, Uno sprinted across the ring as soon as the bell rang. He leaped in the air and tried to connect a flying kick to Penn's face. But Penn brushed it aside, and advanced toward his opponent. Only seven seconds into the fight, Penn landed a left jab on the chin of Uno, twisting Uno's head rapidly to his left. Caol Uno stumbled backward, dazed, disoriented, off-balance, stunned. He fell to the canvas where Penn unleashed a flurry of powerful rights to Uno's face until referee Larry Landless was forced to jump in and end the fight, a mere 10 seconds after it started.

Caol Uno was concussed.

Many readers will have seen similar knockouts during boxing or mixed martial arts bouts. But few will know what happens after the match. Few will know how a concussion should be responded to medically. Few will know what to do if a concussion occurs.

This chapter discusses an ideal approach to the assessment and management of sport-related concussions. It will review several different methods of evaluation and all the facets of care for an injured athlete. No program, physician, or clinic will employ all of these resources, as many are simply different ways of doing the same thing. Only certain methods may be used by your caregivers depending on the risk of concussion in a given sport, the available team resources, the knowledge and skill of personnel caring for athletes, and other factors. Often, medical personnel will use only some of these methods of evaluating athletes who have sustained concussions. For most concussions, which resolve readily without intervention, minimal therapy is all that will be required. Athletes who have more significant symptoms or longer recovery times may be referred to a specialty concussion clinic where a more complete evaluation may be performed and further therapies may be offered.

The assessment and management of concussion starts even before the first game of the season. Several measures, which can later be used to assess a potential injury, can be employed at the start of the season, before the athletes are at risk of sustaining a concussion.

It can be difficult for an athletic trainer or team physician to determine whether an athlete has sustained a concussion. Athletes often do not report their concussions to anyone. Some even downplay about their symptoms when asked. In fact, a study of high school athletes conducted in 2004 by neuropsychologist Michael McCrea revealed that less than half of concussed athletes reported their injury. Although more recent studies suggest that the reporting of concussion has increased among high school athletes, a substantial proportion still do not report their symptoms to anyone. There are various reasons for this. Many do not recognize that their symptoms are due to a concussion. Even those who are knocked unconscious do not always recognize they have sustained a concussion. Many do not realize that a concussion is an injury to the brain. Since symptom reporting is a major part of diagnosing and managing a concussion, the lack of reporting makes it difficult for medical personnel to properly manage sport-related concussions. In order to help determine whether an athlete has sustained a concussion, athletic trainers or team physicians will often perform assessments of symptoms, balance, and brain function before the start of the season. These assessments can then be repeated in the event of a suspected concussion in order to assist these clinicians in making the diagnosis. They can be repeated further to help monitor recovery.

Most sport-related concussion protocols will include the following assessments prior to the start of the season:

1. A symptom inventory
2. A balance assessment
3. A sideline concussion assessment tool
4. A neuropsychological assessment

Each of these is discussed further in the following sections.

SYMPTOM INVENTORIES

A symptom inventory is a measurement of the symptoms most often experienced by athletes after suffering a concussion. The most common symptom after a concussion is headache. Other common symptoms include insomnia, dizziness, amnesia, confusion, difficulty with memory, and difficulty concentrating. Table 7.1, shown later in this chapter, contains many of the symptoms associated with concussion. This will often be collected at the beginning of the season. It can be used in two ways. Some clinicians will ask athletes to report any symptoms they are having at the time of their baseline assessment. Thus, if they had a headache, or were light-headed at the time of the baseline, they would record these symptoms. Other clinicians ask athletes to only record those symptoms that are due to a concussion. Thus, all athletes who were not recovering from a concussion at the time of their baseline assessment would rate a zero for all symptoms. Athletes asked to fill out a symptom inventory, should follow the instructions of the person administering it.

Although many symptom inventories exist, most are similar. Figure 7.1 is an example of the symptom inventory we use at the Sports Concussion Clinic in the Division of Sports Medicine at Children's Hospital Boston. It is based on the post-concussion symptom scale developed by the international conferences on concussion in sports.

Figure 7.1
Symptom Scale (Used by permission)

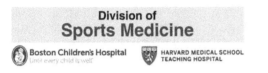

Division of Sports Medicine	Patient label
Boston Children's Hospital — Until every child is well HARVARD MEDICAL SCHOOL TEACHING HOSPITAL	NEW INJURY

Please circle only those symptoms that WERE NOT THERE BEFORE you got your concussion, and are STILL bothering you in the last 24 HOURS

If you have always had a certain symptom, like trouble paying attention, and it is the same as always, then circle 0. But if it is worse than normal choose 1 to 6.

(Please choose only ONE number for each symptom.)

Somatic Symptoms	None	Mild		Moderate		Severe	
Headache	0	1	2	3	4	5	6
"Pressure in head"	0	1	2	3	4	5	6
Neck pain	0	1	2	3	4	5	6
Nausea or vomiting	0	1	2	3	4	5	6
Sensitivity to light	0	1	2	3	4	5	6
Sensitivity to noise	0	1	2	3	4	5	6

Vestibular Symptoms	None	Mild		Moderate		Severe	
Balance problems	0	1	2	3	4	5	6
Dizziness	0	1	2	3	4	5	6
Blurred vision	0	1	2	3	4	5	6

Emotional Symptoms	None	Mild		Moderate		Severe	
More emotional	0	1	2	3	4	5	6
Irritability	0	1	2	3	4	5	6
Sadness	0	1	2	3	4	5	6
Nervous or anxious	0	1	2	3	4	5	6

Cognitive Symptoms	None	Mild		Moderate		Severe	
Confusion	0	1	2	3	4	5	6
Feeling like "in a fog"	0	1	2	3	4	5	6
Difficulty concentrating	0	1	2	3	4	5	6
Difficulty remembering	0	1	2	3	4	5	6
"Don't feel right"	0	1	2	3	4	5	6
Feeling slowed down	0	1	2	3	4	5	6

Sleep Symptoms	None	Mild		Moderate		Severe	
Drowsiness	0	1	2	3	4	5	6
Fatigue or low energy	0	1	2	3	4	5	6
Trouble falling asleep	0	1	2	3	4	5	6

Total PCSS: _____

BALANCE ASSESSMENT

There are several ways to perform balance assessments. Perhaps the easiest and most available method was described by the Third International Consensus on Concussion in Sports. It is a modified version of the balance error scoring system developed by athletic trainer Kevin Guskiewicz and his colleagues. In order to perform the assessment, the examiner needs to have a stopwatch. Athletes are asked to perform three specific stances for 20 seconds each. Athletes should remove shoes, athletic taping, ankle braces, etc., prior to the start of the test.

The first stance requires athletes to stand with their hands on their hips, their feet together, and their eyes closed. The second stance requires athletes to stand on their nondominant foot. The dominant foot is the foot generally used to kick a ball. The opposite foot is known as the nondominant foot. Since my preferred foot for kicking a ball is my right foot, my nondominant foot would be my left one. Again, athletes must have their hands on their hips, their eyes closed, and must hold the stance steady for 20 seconds. The third and final stance requires athletes to stand with one foot in front of the other. In this position, the nondominant foot is placed behind the dominant foot. Once again, athletes must place their hands on their hips, close their eyes and hold the stance for 20 seconds.

During each of three 20-second trials, an error is recorded for athletes if:

1. Their hands are taken off of their hips.
2. They open their eyes.
3. They take a step, stumble or fall.
4. They move their hip too far to one side.
5. They lift their toes or heel off of the ground.
6. They remain out of the stance for more than five seconds.

The total number of errors per trial is recorded, with the maximum allotted number of errors per stance being 10. The official balance examination score is 30 minus the number of errors recorded. For example, if an athlete has impeccable balance, and does not commit any errors, he would score a perfect 30. If another athlete opened her eyes during the first stance, stumbled during the second stance, lifted her heel off the ground later in the second stance, and performed perfectly in the third stance, she would have committed three total errors. Her final balance examination score would be 27.

There are other ways of assessing balance. Several machines can measure the amount of sway or rocking a person does when standing in certain positions. But these machines and the associated computer software can be fairly expensive. Often these are cost prohibitive for smaller, less well funded athletic programs. Even a television video game device known as the Wii Fit can be used to assess balance. In fact, the Wii Fit has even made its way into the medical literature in this regard. But currently, the modified Balance Error Scoring System is the most thoroughly studied, most easily understood, and most readily available for use in managing sport-related concussions. It is best used, by obtaining a baseline BESS score, prior to the start of the season, when an athlete is healthy. Then, repeated scores after a concussion can be used to monitor recovery.

Sideline Concussion Assessment Tools

It can often be unclear when a concussion has occurred. Athletes do not always recognize the signs and symptoms of concussion. Even when they know they have sustained a concussion, they are often reluctant to report it for fear of losing playing time, their position on the team, the respect of their teammates, the respect of their coach, their reputation for toughness, and various other reasons. Even when athletes report signs and symptoms such as headaches, lightheadedness and poor balance during a game, it can be difficult sometimes to tell whether the athlete has sustained a concussion or the symptoms are due to something else, like dehydration. Sideline concussion assessment tools were developed in order to assist on-site medical personnel in diagnosing a sport-related concussion. They are intended to be used at the sideline or rink side during practice or competition when an athlete is suspected of having sustained a sport-related concussion. During practice and game times, athletes are often tired, sweaty, dehydrated and distracted. Therefore, the best time to perform baseline sideline concussion assessments is in the middle or near the end of a practice. This helps account somewhat for these factors. There are several standardized sideline concussion assessment tools. We will discuss some of the more commonly used versions in the following sections.

The Maddocks Questions

Many readers will recall being struck in the head during athletics when they were younger. If you received any medical attention at all, it was likely a concerned parent, coach, or, if you were lucky, an athletic trainer. I remember this from when I was a kid. They might shine a light in your eyes. They might ask you your name, where you were, what day of the week it was, what time it was, or who the president was. These types of questions were designed to determine whether the athlete was "oriented" to person (who he or she was), place (where he or she was) and time (what day of the week and time of day it was). These were not difficult questions to answer, even for players who were concussed. Furthermore, the answers mattered little. Even when you got them wrong, people simply laughed and had you rest for a while, only to be returned to your sport later on that same day. At the time, concussion was not thought to be an injury of any consequence.

As we learned more about concussions, about the potential for complications after a concussion, about prolonged recoveries from concussions and about the potential long-term effects of sustaining multiple concussions, sports medicine personnel started to develop better ways for determining whether an athlete had sustained a sport-related concussion. In 1995, a man named David Maddocks out of the University of Melbourne in Australia compared the answers to these questions, which assessed orientation, to the answers of questions regarding more immediate memory. His study was conducted on Australian rules football players who had sustained a concussion. Specifically, the questions he used to judge recent memory were:

1. At which ground are we (playing)?
2. Which quarter is it?
3. How far into the quarter is it—first, middle or last 10 minutes?
4. Which side kicked the last goal?
5. Which team did we play last week?
6. Did we win last week?

He found that concussed athletes found these questions pertaining to recent memory more difficult to answer than the questions used to determine general orientation. These questions have since come to be known as the "Maddocks" questions. They must be tailored for other sports. For example, to use them during an ice hockey match, one would have to replace "quarter" with "period." They are currently used by many sports medicine clinicians to help determine when an athlete has sustained a concussion.

They are included in the sport concussion assessment tool version 5 (SCAT 5) discussed further later.

Standardized Assessment of Concussion (SAC)

The standardized assessment of concussion (SAC) was developed by a neuropsychologist named Michael McCrea. This sideline assessment has several components. It consists of four main components, used to assess: orientation, immediate memory, concentration, and delayed recall (delayed memory). The general orientation component assesses whether the athlete is able to recall the month, date, day of the week, year and approximate time of day. In the assessment of immediate memory, athletes are asked to recall a list of five words that were given to them by the examiner. While assessing concentration, athletes are asked to perform certain tasks, such as repeating a string of digits given to them by the examiner in reverse order. Reciting the months of the year in reverse order is another task for assessing concentration. In the delayed memory section, athletes are asked to recall the five words they were given previously. Each section is scored. The scores from each section are summed to give a total score. The test is meant to be performed at the start of the season. The preseason score serves as a baseline. Athletes suspected of having sustained a concussion repeat the test. Their post-injury score is then compared to their preseason baseline score.

Like all sideline assessment tools, the SAC is meant to be performed during a practice or competition in the event of a suspected concussion. Therefore, baseline scores should be obtained in similar circumstances, when an athlete has been working out and may be tired, may be mildly dehydrated, or may have decreased energy reserves, in order to simulate the state during competition and practice. Like the Maddocks questions, the SAC has also been incorporated into SCAT 5, which is discussed further next.

Sport Concussion Assessment Tool (SCAT 5)

In 2004 a group of sport-related concussion experts met in Prague, Czech Republic, to "provide recommendations for the improvement of safety and health of athletes who suffer concussive brain injuries." In the summary and agreement statement from this meeting, the sport concussion assessment tool (SCAT) was published. It was developed by combining aspects of previous existing tools. The same group met again every four years since and repeatedly updated the tool, publishing the most recent version, SCAT 5. The SCAT 5 contains the SAC and the Maddocks questions, discussed earlier, within it. It is available for free on the World Wide Web. It is not subject to copyright restrictions. It is designed to be used by medical and health professionals.

The SCAT 5 is the longest and most comprehensive of the sideline assessments. As noted, it incorporates several of the other available sideline assessments into it. It starts with a symptom inventory. It takes into account whether the athlete had gross imbalance or a loss of consciousness. It includes the Glasgow coma scale discussed in Chapter 18 of this book, which is not useful for predicting recovery or long-term effects from concussion, but his highly useful in the immediate assessment of an acutely injured athlete. It includes both the Maddocks questions and SAC discussed earlier. It includes the modified Balance Error Scoring System and some well-known neurological tests of physical coordination. The numbers of points athletes score on each section are added to yield a total, which can be compared to baseline scores. Finally, the SCAT 5 concludes with a summary and advice that can be given to the athlete. While these sideline assessment tools help medical personnel assess potential sport-related concussions, they are not used alone. A medical history, a physical examination, a symptom inventory, a sideline assessment, a balance assessment and computerized neuropsychological testing should all be incorporated into a detailed concussion assessment and management protocol.

Often, sports medicine professionals will also ask athletes about their "concussion history," prior to the start of the season. A concussion history is a summary of any previous concussions, in or outside of sports that the athlete has sustained. How many concussions the athlete has sustained, how long it took the athlete to recover from each, how each concussion occurred, when each concussion occurred, how significant the signs and symptoms of concussion were after each injury, are all important details that will be used to determine management of future sport-related concussions. Many times, this concussion history will be obtained as part of the overall pre-participation physical examination.

Finally, a neuropsychological assessment should be performed on athletes prior to the start of the season. Although many sideline assessments include some neuropsychological tests as one of their components, these tests are brief and, at times, cursory. They consist of large or gross assessments of brain function. Many athletes, even after sustaining a sport-related concussion, will be able to perform the tasks required by these sideline assessments prior to being fully recovered. Therefore, more complete and thorough neuropsychological tests should be performed prior to the start of the season. Most often, these will be computerized neurocognitive assessments. Currently, there are several computerized neurocognitive assessments available for purchase. So, we now know some of the assessments and measurements that will be performed prior to the start of the season. These can be used to diagnose a concussion or monitor an athlete's recovery after a concussion. Let us now discuss what may happen when a concussion occurs.

Concussion is the most common brain injury in sports. But it is not the only one. Athletes can sustain skull fractures, often with bleeding in and around the brain. Even without a skull fracture athletes can suffer bleeding in and around the brain. They can suffer swelling of the brain. They can sustain a bruise of the brain. They can sustain a neck injury, including fractures of the cervical spine, which is the portion of the spine contained within the neck. Fractures of the cervical spine can be associated with damage to the spinal cord. Therefore, when an athlete sustains an injury to the head, the first concern of the medical team is not whether the athlete has a concussion. More immediate, time-sensitive issues need to be assessed for, evaluated, and treated, before consideration of a concussion.

All personnel in the medical field are trained to respond to an acute injury in an organized fashion. The most pressing, emergent potential issues are assessed and treated immediately. Once all life-threatening issues have been addressed, the assessment continues, often focusing on less emergent injuries. An easy way clinicians use to remember the start of the emergency response is "A B C."

"A" stands for airway. When medical personnel arrive at the scene of an acutely injured athlete, the first task is to assess the airway. This means making sure that the mouth of the patient is open, and that nothing is blocking the flow of air from the mouth to the lungs. This is particularly important in an athlete who has sustained a head injury. When athletes are knocked unconscious, especially if they are lying on their backs, their tongue, tonsils, soft palate, other structures in the mouth, as well as object such as tobacco products, chewing gum, teeth knocked loose at the time of impact, or mouth guards, may move to the back of the throat. These tissues and objects can block the flow of air from the mouth and nose to the lungs. This will prevent the patient from breathing. These tissues and objects must be cleared away from the airway, in order for the patient to breathe. As a result, you may see the athletic trainer, team physician, emergency medical technician or other medical response personnel remove the mouth guard, remove any other objects in the mouth, and position the patient's jaw in such a way that air can flow freely to the lungs.

For readers who have taken courses in first aid, wilderness medicine or cardiopulmonary resuscitation (CPR), this may sound familiar. You may even recall some of the skills you were taught to reposition the airway. One of the more common is called the chin-lift maneuver. However, when an athlete is unconscious after an injury to the head, we do not perform the chin-lift maneuver. The chin-lift maneuver results in movement of the cervical spine. When athletes are unconscious after a blow to the head, they may have also injured or fractured their cervical spine. When the cervical spine is fractured, any inappropriate movement of the neck may make the fracture worse, and may result in damage to the spinal cord. Therefore, methods for clearing the airway that do not result in movement of the neck and cervical spine are preferred. Most commonly, the jaw-thrust technique is used.

In order to perform the jaw thrust maneuver, medical responders place their fingers behind the jaw bone, just underneath the ear lobes. The jaw is then pushed forward, such that the lower teeth move forward. The tongue and other tissues are brought forward with the jaw, thus clearing them from the airway, allowing air to pass through to the lungs, with minimal associated movement of the neck. Although this looks awkward and uncomfortable for the patient, it is a life-saving maneuver. It is important that parents, coaches, teammates and other caring spectators allow the medical team to do their work, without interfering. Any attempts to stop or interfere with the medical responders can result in catastrophic outcomes, including death and paralysis.

"B" is for breathing. Once the airway has been cleared of the tongue, other tissues, and other objects, the medical responder will make sure that the patient is breathing. Breathing is most often assessed by:

1. Looking to see if the patient's chest is rising and falling as it typically does when a person breathes.
2. Listening for the sounds made in the chest when a person breathes. This may be accomplished by placing a stethoscope on the athlete's chest or by simply placing an ear directly against the athlete's chest.
3. Feeling for the rise and fall of the chest. This is most often accomplished by the medical responder resting his or her hand on the athlete's chest.
4. Feeling for the flow of air from the mouth. This can be accomplished by the medical responder placing his or her hand or cheek in front of the mouth and nose of the injured athlete.

If the athlete is not breathing, the medical responder will assist the patient with breathing. Again, there are several ways of doing this. One way is by giving rescue breaths or mouth-to-mouth resuscitation, where the medical responder seals his or her mouth with that of the athlete and blows air into the injured athlete's mouth, through the throat, and into the lungs. More commonly, the medical responder will place a mask over the mouth of the athlete. This mask is attached to a bag of air. When the bag is squeezed, air from inside the bag travels through the mask, into the patient's mouth, through the throat, and into the lungs.

Once the athlete is breathing, the medical responder will proceed to "C."

"C" is for circulation. Once it has been determined that an athlete's airway is clear and the athlete is breathing, the medical responder will assess for a heartbeat. This is most often accomplished by feeling for a pulse, either in the athlete's wrist or neck. If there is no pulse, the responder will try to pump blood from the heart to the rest of the body by performing "chest compressions." During chest compressions, the responder will apply pressure to the heart by pushing the portion of the athlete's chest that lies directly over the heart down one or two inches. This pressure is then released by letting go of the chest. When the heart is squeezed like this repeatedly, blood flows out of the heart, through the arteries, and supplies blood to the remainder of the body, including the brain. Again, it should be emphasized that while this appears awkward and uncomfortable for the athlete, it is a potentially life-saving technique. Spectators must not interfere with emergency responders during one of these situations.

It should be noted, that recent changes in these techniques have focused less on assisting breathing, and more on performing chest compressions to assist with circulation. The order of these responses may differ, depending on the current recommendations, the skills of the responder, the number of medical personnel available, and the immediate needs of the athlete.

Although this assessment and resuscitation strategies can seem complex when reading about them, they can be performed quickly by trained and experienced personnel. In an athlete who is conscious, the airway, breathing and circulation can be assessed simply by asking an athlete, "how are you?" If the athlete answers, then the medical responder knows that the airway is open, the athlete is breathing, and the heart is beating. Therefore, the remainder of the assessment can begin.

The remainder of the assessment after trauma is detailed and can seem complex to those unfamiliar with medical terminology and procedure. For the reader who is not medically trained, it would require an extensive discussion. Therefore, it is not included here. For those interested in learning more about the medical response to trauma, several articles and books are available and included in the suggested readings section at the end of this chapter.

A NOTE TO THE MEDICALLY TRAINED: For those readers who have taken courses in cardiopulmonary resuscitation or other medical interventions I would like to add a word of caution. Many athletic events will have medical personnel on the scene. These medical professionals will be well-trained in the assessment and management of patients who sustain trauma. In addition, those who routinely cover these events will be well-trained and knowledgeable about the unique injuries sustained by athletes and the unique techniques that must be used to assess and manage athletes. The response to trauma and resuscitation of athletes differs in several ways from the response to and resuscitation of other patients. In particular, athletes wearing bulky padding and athletic equipment must be managed according to different protocols than nonathletes who sustain trauma. If such medical personnel are present, it is best to allow them to do their work without interfering. Many spectators who are medically trained will want to help or assist in these situations. Unless they have particular experience in the response to an injured athlete, however, they are more likely to cause harm than to be helpful.

A NOTE ABOUT NECK AND CERVICAL SPINE INJURIES: As mentioned previously, the "cervical spine" refers to the bones of the spine that reside within the neck. Nerves cells originating in the brain travel through the neck, forming what is known as the spinal cord. The spinal cord descends from the brain through the neck and down the back. It sends nerves to the various parts of the body. Fractures and other injuries to the cervical spine can damage the spinal cord, resulting in serious, permanent neurological injury. Athletes who sustain fractures and other injuries to the cervical spine, can suffer permanent paralysis or even death. Therefore, the medical response team takes great care to avoid unnecessary movement of the neck while responding to and resuscitating an injured athlete. This concern is heightened in the athlete who sustained a sport related concussion associated with a change in mental status, confusion, or loss of consciousness.

Many times, however, an athlete who sustains a blow to the head experiences more subtle signs or symptoms. It is clear early in the evaluation that there are no signs or symptoms of bleeding in the brain, cervical spine injury, swelling of the brain or other emergent issues. The medical responder focuses on whether the athlete has sustained a concussion. Often, it is obvious that the player has sustained a concussion. But sometimes it can be more subtle. The medical team may use some of the preseason assessments discussed earlier, to decide whether an athlete has sustained a concussion.

In a conscious athlete, medical personnel will often start by determining whether the athlete is oriented. As described previously, the term "orientation" refers to a person's understanding of his or her current surroundings and circumstances, often focusing on person, place and time: Do the athletes know 1) who they are, 2) where they are and 3) what time of day, week, month, or year it is? In order to test an athlete's "orientation," medical personnel often ask some basic questions such as:

- What is your name?
- Where are you right now?
- What time of day is it?
- What day of the week is it?
- What is today's date?
- Who is the president of the United States?

This gives on site medical personnel an immediate, but very broad, general insight into an injured athlete's brain functioning. Failure to answer these basic questions correctly can be a sign of serious injury, and will often prompt a more urgent medical response. If an athlete is oriented, the medical responder will often assess for the signs and symptoms of concussion. As a review, the signs and symptoms of concussion are listed in Tables 7.1 and 7.2. Remember, the word "symptoms" refers to the characteristics of illness that are felt or experienced by the patient. Things like headache, nausea, feeling "out of it," and sensitivity to light are all *symptoms* of a concussion. The word "signs" refers to the characteristics of illness that can be seen by those observing the patients. Unconsciousness, disorientation, confusion, and poor balance are all *signs* of a concussion.

Table 7.1
Common Symptoms of a Sport-Related Concussion

Symptoms of Concussion

- Headache
- Dizziness
- Difficulty concentrating
- Nausea or vomiting
- Difficulty balancing
- Vision changes
- Sensitivity to light
- Sensitivity to noise
- Feeling "out of it"
- Ringing in the ears
- Drowsiness
- Sadness

Table 7.2
Common Signs of a Sport-Related Concussion

Signs of Concussion

- Loss of consciousness
- Amnesia, or forgetfulness
- Walking off-balance
- Acting disoriented
- Appearing dazed
- Acting confused
- Forgetting game rules or play assignments
- Inability to recall score or opponent
- Inappropriate emotionality
- Poor physical coordination
- Slow verbal responses
- Personality changes

By looking at these tables, one can see that many of the signs and symptoms of concussion are associated with other illnesses or medical conditions. Dehydration, which is common during athletic competition, can cause headaches, dizziness, and sensitivity to light. In order to help distinguish whether an athlete's signs and symptoms are due to concussion versus some other medical condition, medical personnel will often focus on the facts surrounding the onset of symptoms. For example, if an athlete skates off of the ice during a hockey game and tells the athletic trainer he feels light-headed and has a headache, the athletic trainer will often ask the athlete a series of questions:

1. When did the headache start?
2. Did it come on gradually or did it start suddenly?
3. Were you struck in the head at the time the headache started?
4. Do you feel nauseous?
5. Have you ever felt this way before?
6. How did you feel before the game started?

The answers to these initial questions will often lead to other questions. The object is to get a full understanding of how the symptoms started, and how they have the changed since they started. For example, the athlete may report that he awoke late for class that day and skipped breakfast. He had a chicken sandwich for lunch without a drink. He was mildly lightheaded when he stood up initially for his line change during the first period. He noticed a small headache during the intermission between first and second period. It has since progressed. He has not sustained any major body checks or blows to the head.

In this case, the athletic trainer may conclude the athlete is likely dehydrated. He may be offered a sports drink or even intravenous fluids. He may be allowed to continue playing.

Alternatively, the athlete may report that he felt well all game until he sustained an open ice body check that lifted him off of his feet, causing him to land head first on the ice. He experienced the immediate onset of headaches. He rose up to finish the play and noticed he was light-headed for the first time that day. He skated off the ice and reported to the athletic trainer.

In this case, the athletic trainer might conclude that the athlete has sustained a concussion. He would be removed from play and further assessment would begin.

Typically, medical personnel will assess for signs and symptoms of other potential injuries discussed previously, such as bleeding in or around the brain, swelling of the brain, and neck or cervical spine injury. If there were no other injuries, then medical personnel might use one of the symptoms inventories or sideline assessments discussed earlier to help decide whether an athlete has sustained a concussion. Sometimes, this will be unnecessary, as the diagnosis can be made without the use of these preseason evaluations.

Once the diagnosis of concussion has been made, the athlete should be removed from play immediately. Continuing to play with a concussion places the athlete at risk for a prolonged recovery, more pronounced deficits in brain functioning, and catastrophic injuries such as second impact syndrome.

Once concussed athletes have been removed from play, they should be monitored for the next few hours. As was mentioned earlier, concussion is the most common neurological injury in sports. But it is not the only one. Swelling of the brain, bleeding into or around the brain, and bruising of the brain may not always be apparent immediately after injury. Occasionally, more extensive damage to the brain will not be detectable or obvious until minutes to hours later. Therefore, athletes who have sustained a suspected sport-related concussion should be observed closely and monitored, with someone checking on them every 15 to 20 minutes for the first few hours after injury. Often, these neurological checks will be performed by the athletic trainer or team physician while the athlete remains at the field side, rink side, or arena. However, when the contest is over and all athletes are leaving the area of play, others may be asked to perform monitoring and observation of the athlete. Teammates, roommates, family members, and others should be asked to monitor the patient over the first 24 hours. Any concerning signs or symptoms should prompt the athlete to seek emergency medical attention.

Some of the signs and symptoms of more extensive brain injury are:

- Persistent vomiting or the new onset of vomiting
- Somnolence, where the athlete appears sleepy and is difficult to rouse
- Persistent confusion, disorientation or the new onset of confusion or disorientation
- Seizure
- Appearing abnormal

Although "appearing abnormal" is a vague phrase, it is meant to be so. It can be difficult to describe exactly what it is abnormal about a traumatically brain injured athlete. But most people can tell when something is wrong. Most people have an intuitive sense, an innate ability, to determine sick from nonsick, worrisome from not worrisome. If ever you get the sense that something is concerning about an athlete suspected of having sustained a sport-related concussion, seek immediate medical attention. It is better to raise the alarm and find out later that the athlete has a concussion from which he or she will recover completely, then to miss a potentially catastrophic brain injury.

Athletes will recover from concussions spontaneously. At present, there is no medication or other therapy that is proven to treat concussion. However, there are some steps athletes can take to avoid worsening of their symptoms and, perhaps, to help them recover faster.

Physical rest: After athletes sustain a concussion, they are immediately removed from sports so that they won't hit their heads again, and sustain another concussion. However, there is another reason for removing the athlete from sport. For many athletes, physical exertion makes their symptoms worse, particularly during the first few days after injury. Even noncontact activities such as running, ice skating, weight lifting, and working out on exercise machines, will often make symptoms worse. So as soon as an athlete has been diagnosed with a concussion, he or she should be removed from all forms of training and exercise for the first few days. This will treat the symptoms and, perhaps, help athletes to recover faster.

Cognitive rest: The Merriam-Webster dictionary defines cognitive as "of, relating to, being, or involving conscious intellectual activity (as thinking, reasoning, or remembering)." Cognitive processes are those that involve thinking, remembering, concentrating, or reasoning. Cognitive rest requires avoiding cognitive activities such as reading, writing, doing homework, playing games such as chess or Trivial Pursuit, playing video games, text messaging, working online, and so forth. Often the symptoms of an athlete recovering from a concussion will get worse during these activities, particularly during the first few days after injury. Athletes should be encouraged to avoid cognitive activities during the first few days of recovery from a sport-related concussion. For student athletes, this can be quite difficult. When in school, an athlete is required to perform cognitive activities on a daily basis. Nearly all schoolwork requires reading, writing, reasoning, remembering and concentrating. Therefore, I often recommend athletes stay home from school for a few days immediately following a sport-related concussion, if they are experiencing symptoms. While missing school is never ideal, students will miss school on various occasions such, when they have the flu, when they are vomiting, when a parent takes them on a vacation, and for many other reasons. Certainly, missing a few days of school in order to recover from a traumatic brain injury is warranted. I recommend no more than 2–3 days of absence from school. Many athletes will be fully or nearly symptom-free at that point. In fact, nearly 85 percent of high school athletes report being completely symptom free and are deemed by their athletic trainer to be recovered within one week after their injury. The time until recovery is even shorter for older athletes. Concussed athletes will note significant improvement in their symptoms after the first several days if they truly rest themselves, avoiding both physical and cognitive exertion. Therefore, no other treatments will be necessary to treat the majority of sport-related concussions.

Steps to take if you suspect an athlete has sustained a sport-related concussion:

1. Remove the athlete from play immediately.
2. Take the athlete directly to on-site medical personnel so they can evaluate the athlete, check for other potential injuries, administer any needed treatments, and instruct you further.
3. If there is no on-site medical personnel, take the athlete to a doctor, or, if necessary, call for an ambulance.
4. If medical personnel diagnose the athlete with a concussion, check on the athlete every 15–20 minutes for the first few hours after injury. If you see anything concerning, call a doctor or, if necessary, an ambulance.

5. Encourage physical and cognitive rest as described earlier. This should start immediately and should include an absence from school for the first few days if the athlete is not feeling better.
6. Schedule an appointment with the athlete's primary care physician, or, if the athlete has already been diagnosed with a concussion as opposed to another illness or injury, a clinician with experience in the assessment and management of sport-related concussions.

In order to help illustrate some of these points, an example of how an acutely injured athlete might be evaluated and managed on site is provided here.

Kevin is a 15-year-old football player for a local high school. Although only a sophomore, he is both fast and strong for his age. He often plays with the varsity football team. It is late in the third quarter. Kevin's team is winning by three points. He has been playing on both sides of the ball, participating in both offense and defense. Currently, his team is on offense. They have driven down the field to his opponents' 17-yard line. As Kevin is the strongest running back on the team, the coach puts him in. It's third down. They need a total of four yards to get another first down. The ball is snapped. The quarterback turns to his left and fakes a hand-off to the halfback. He then pitches back to Kevin. Kevin takes the ball, lowers his shoulder, and follows the halfback toward the defensive line. The halfback attempts to block one of the oncoming defenseman. However, he is run down and Kevin is struck simultaneously by two on-rushing defenders. Kevin's helmet collides with that of one of his opponents. He is knocked backward to the ground. The back of his head bounces off the turf.

Kevin's teammates immediately realize something is wrong. He is not moving on the ground. He makes no effort to stand up. They rush to his side and frantically wave for the coach and athletic trainer to come on to the field. When the athletic trainer arrives, he sees that Kevin is lying on the ground motionless not responding to his name. The athletic trainer sends two of the other players and one of the assistant coaches to call for an ambulance.

Immediately the athletic trainer takes what looks like a pair of pliers from his bag. He cuts the two rubber bands on the side of Kevin's helmet that hold the face mask in place. He removes the face mask from the helmet and puts it aside. He removes Kevin's mouth guard, and opens his mouth. Seeing that there are no other objects in Kevin's mouth, he listens to see whether Kevin is breathing. However he is unable to hear Kevin's breath sounds through his jersey, shoulder pads, and breastplate. He quickly removes a pair of scissors from his medical bag. He cuts Kevin's jersey straight down the middle and down each of the sleeves. He cuts the laces at the center of Kevin's breastplate as well as the straps around his arms. He opens the breastplate, exposing Kevin's chest. He places his ear on the chest and is able to hear Kevin breathing both on the right and left sides of his chest. He sees that Kevin's chest rises on both the left and right sides. He then holds Kevin by the wrist, feeling for a pulse, which he notes is present and strong. He moves to Kevin's head, grasps his helmet on either side, and prevents any movement of Kevin's head and neck.

Two additional athletic trainers arrive around the same time as the ambulance. The emergency medical technicians place a large plastic board at Kevin's side. The emergency medical technicians and an athletic trainer each line up on Kevin's right side. When the athletic trainer who is holding Kevin's head counts to three, they roll Kevin up on his side. One of the other athletic trainers slides the plastic board up against Kevin's side, in the space where he was just lying. Again, the athletic trainer holding Kevin's head counts to three. They roll him onto his back, such that he is now lying on top of the hard plastic board. They attempt to place a hard plastic collar around Kevin's neck. Realizing that they cannot place the collar safely, because Kevin's helmet and shoulder pads are in the way, they place the collar aside on the ground. Using the previously cut laces of Kevin's breastplate, as well as some athletic tape, they re-secure his shoulder pads to his body. Two padded blocks are placed on either side of Kevin's neck. His helmet, shoulder pads, and the remainder of his body are secured to the hard, plastic board using webbing straps. The board is lifted and placed into the ambulance. Kevin is transported to a local emergency department.

On the way to the hospital, Kevin wakes up. He is clearly anxious and somewhat confused. He does not understand why he is in an ambulance. He is visibly anxious. He continues to ask the ambulance driver where his parents are. He is told multiple times what occurred at the field and that he is on his way to an emergency department. He continues to ask where his parents are. When he arrives in the emergency department Kevin is much calmer. He is still somewhat confused. He is able to tell doctors that he was playing in a football game earlier that day. He does not, however, recall the injury. He does realize he is in an emergency department but cannot recall which city he is in. Ultimately, his football helmet and shoulder pads are removed very carefully by the nurses and doctors in the emergency department, such that they do not cause significant movement of his head or neck. He is placed in a hard plastic collar.

The doctor in the emergency department asks Kevin multiple questions. He spends several minutes examining Kevin and having him perform various tasks. During the examination Kevin's parents arrive. The doctor explains to them that Kevin was injured during the football game. Although he is somewhat disoriented, he otherwise appears well. The doctor tells his parents that as a precaution, they are going to observe him in the emergency department to ensure that he does not have any signs or symptoms of other injuries to the brain or neck. If he develops any concerning signs or symptoms, the doctor explains, they will likely get a picture of Kevin's brain known as a "head CT."

Kevin is admitted to the hospital. Periodically throughout the night nurses and doctors come in and wake Kevin, ask him some questions, and examine him. Over the course of the evening and the following morning he returns back to normal. He is able to answer all questions. He is able to perform all the tasks asked by the doctors examining him. The doctors feel the back of Kevin's neck and ask if he has any pain or tenderness there. He does not. They loosen the collar from around his neck and ask him to slowly move his head in all different directions, instructing him to stop if he develops any pain or unusual sensations. Kevin is able to look all around the room without any difficulty, pain, tenderness, or other unusual sensations. The plastic collar is removed. Although Kevin continues to complain of headaches and difficulty concentrating, he and his parents are informed that this is typical after a concussion. They expect that these symptoms will resolve over the next several days to weeks. They discharge him to home, instructing him to follow up with a specialist in sport-related concussion over the next week or two. They instruct him to avoid all physical activity, exercising, and football until he sees the specialist. The doctors also recommend he avoids school, homework, reading, playing video games, working online and any other forms of cognitive activity.

Several things are worth noting about this example:

1. Once the athletic trainer had access to Kevin and confirmed that (1) his airway was open, (2) he was breathing, and (3) he had a pulse, he immediately focused his attention on ensuring that Kevin's head and neck did not move more than necessary. As discussed previously, injuries to the cervical spine and spinal cord can be devastating. Therefore, this is one of the top priorities of medical personnel responding to an injured athlete once it has been established that the airway is open, the athlete is breathing, and that the athlete has a pulse.

2. When Kevin is placed on the hard plastic board for transport to the emergency department, it is the athletic trainer holding his head and neck in place who controls his movements by directing the rest of the team when and how to move Kevin, and counting to three in order to coordinate the timing of each movement. This is standard medical practice. Since it is of utmost importance to minimize any inappropriate movements of the injured athlete's head and neck, the person controlling the head and neck determines when all movements take place. Typically, the medical provider will instruct the other medical personnel to move the patient in a specific way "on the count of three."

3. Kevin was placed in the ambulance and transported to the emergency department without a hard collar placed on his neck. While this may seem surprising to readers with some medical training, this is the ideal way to transport an athlete with helmets and shoulder pads that inhibit the placement of a hard neck collar. Multiple medical studies have shown that attempting to place a hard neck collar, also known as a cervical collar, on an athlete wearing helmets and shoulder pads can result in significant movement and poor alignment of the bones of the neck. This movement increases the athletes risk for catastrophic outcome such as spinal cord injury. Although there are situations in which the helmets and shoulder pads need to be removed on site, they are rare. When the shoulder pads and helmet need to be removed, then a hard neck collar should be placed. In ideal circumstances, the athlete will be transported wearing the helmet and shoulder pads or there would be sufficient medical personnel with knowledge and experience of equipment removal on site to do it at the field.

4. Kevin did not receive a computed tomogram of the head, more commonly known as a head CT. Many parents, other concerned relatives, and friends of the athlete will want to be absolutely sure that there is no bleeding or swelling of the brain. Many more will be under the impression that a doctor can "see" a concussion on a head CT. Therefore, they will often ask for a head CT. Certainly, many athletes who present to an emergency department after sustaining an injury to the head will require a head CT in order to make sure that there are no such injuries to the brain. However, in order to obtain the pictures of the brain that make up the head CT, radiation is

delivered to the brain. Therefore, a great deal of thought is put into deciding whether an injured athlete requires a head CT. The amount of radiation to which the athlete is exposed during a head CT is a relatively small. Therefore, if the emergency medicine physician treating you or your athlete feels a head CT is warranted, you should not worry about this small amount of radiation. However, if the doctor in the emergency department does not believe a head CT is indicated, then it is better not to have one. The decision to obtain or not obtain a head CT is best left to the doctors examining the injured athlete.

5. When Kevin is discharged from the hospital the doctors who cared for him during his hospital stay instructed him to avoid physical exertion, cognitive exertion, and football, until he is cleared to resume these activities by a physician with expertise in assessing and managing sport-related concussions. This is an ideal situation. However, with the enormous amount of medical literature produced every day, and the speed with which medical recommendations change in response to new discoveries, it is impossible for all physicians to be up to date and well-informed regarding all illnesses and injuries. Therefore, the doctor caring for your athlete may make recommendations based on older medical guidelines. This should not alarm you. This is not reflective of the physician's intelligence or medical capabilities. It simply reflects the rapid speed with which medical science involves and the enormous volumes of information in the medical literature. Doctors need to prioritize those medical issues that are of greatest importance for their practice. For physicians working in the emergency department or in the hospital, it is most important to make sure that any emergent issues are realized and treated. Therefore, this will be the focus of their efforts. This will be the medical literature with which they will be most familiar. After leaving the hospital, you should schedule a follow-up appointment with your primary care physician, a sports medicine physician, or other clinician experienced in the assessment and management of sport-related concussions. These doctors can give you the up to date information on recovering from a sport-related concussion.

In summary, the assessment of sport-related concussion should start prior to the start of the season by obtaining baseline measurements of athletes' symptoms, balance and neurocognitive function. There are several available tools to help clinicians make and record these measurements. When a suspected concussion occurs, the first priority of the responding medical providers is to make sure there are no emergent injuries that require immediate assessment and management. Once any emergent issues have been addressed, medical providers will determine whether a concussion has occurred. Athletes who have sustained a sport-related concussion should be immediately removed from sports and put on both physical and cognitive rest. They should be monitored for the first 24 hours after injury, after injury. Any concerning signs or symptoms should result in immediate medical attention. Most athletes will recover from a sport-related concussion quickly, within days to weeks, requiring only physical and cognitive rest for the first few days in order to fully recover.

SUGGESTED READINGS

American College of Surgeons. *Advanced Trauma Life Support for Doctors, Student Manual*, 8th Edition. Chicago: American College of Surgeons, 2008.

Banerjee, R., M. A. Palumbo, and P. D. Fadale. Catastrophic cervical spine injuries in the collision sport athlete, Part 2: Principles of emergency care. *Am J Sports Med*, 2004, 32(7): 1760–1764.

Concussion (mild traumatic brain injury) and the team physician: A consensus statement. *Med Sci Sports Exerc*, 2006, 38(2): 395–399.

Guskiewicz, K. M., S. E. Ross, and S. W. Marshall. Postural stability and neuropsychological deficits after concussion in collegiate athletes. *J Athl Train*, 2001, 36(3): 263–273.

Harris, M. B., and R. K. Sethi. The initial assessment and management of the multiple-trauma patient with an associated spine injury. *Spine* (Phila Pa 1976), 2006, 31(11 Suppl): S9–S15; discussion S36.

Howell, D. R., et al. Physical activity level and symptom duration are not associated after concussion. *Am J Sports Med*, 2016, 44(4): 1040–1046.

LaRoche, A. A., L. D. Nelson, P. K. Conelly, K. D. Walter, M. A. McCrea. Sport-related concussion reporting and state legislative effects. *Clin J Sport Med*, 2016, 26(1): 33–39.

McCrea, M., et al. Standardized assessment of concussion in football players. *Neurology*, 1997, 48(3): 586–588.

McCrea, M., et al. Unreported concussion in high school football players: Implications for prevention. *Clin J Sport Med*, 2004, 14(1): 13–17.

McCrory, P., et al. Consensus statement on concussion in sport: The Fifth International Conference on Concussion in Sport held in Berlin, October 2016. *Br J Sports Med*, 2017 [Epub ahead of print].

Swartz, E. E., et al. National athletic trainers' association position statement: Acute management of the cervical spine-injured athlete. *J Athl Train*, 2009, 44(3): 306–331.

8

POTENTIAL THERAPIES: WHAT CAN BE DONE TO HELP AN ATHLETE RECOVER

On May 26, 2010, the Boston Celtics were playing the Orlando magic in game 5 of the Eastern Conference finals. Dwight Howard pulled up for a shot. As he descended, his left elbow struck the Celtics forward Glen "Big Baby" Davis in the face. Davis lay on the ground for several seconds, staring into space. His first attempt to stand resulted in his simply lifting his head and shoulders up, only to relax back shortly. The second time he attempted to stand, he scurried along on all fours, unable to get his feet underneath his large, powerful frame. When he was finally able to get to his feet, he stumbled off to his left, visibly off-balance, away from the play, until he collapsed into the arms of the official. His teammates came to support him. But he was so unsteady on his feet that he ultimately was placed on the ground to be assessed by the team's sports medicine staff.

Glen Davis was concussed.

As with most concussed athletes, Glen Davis was prescribed physical rest, which kept him from sustaining another injury to the head, and may have hastened his recovery.

While most athletes will recover quickly from their sport-related concussions, some will have a more prolonged recovery period. Approximately 2 percent of high school athletes who sustain a sport-related concussion will have symptoms that last longer than a month. For some of these athletes, it will be many months or even up to a year until their symptoms resolved. For this unfortunate minority, there are many other considerations.

PHYSICAL REST

As outlined, physical rest is recommendations given to concussed athletes in order to help them feel better and recovery more quickly. Avoiding physical activity for the first several days is usually not much of an issue or challenge.

Athletes who are in school must be excused from gym class. This will often require a note from a physician. If possible, recess should be allowed, but monitored, so that the athlete is safe, without an increased risk of trauma to the head or overexertion leading to an exacerbation of symptoms. Under no circumstances should athletes be cleared for return to contact or collision sports before they are completely recovered from their concussions. The duration for which physical rest is recommended, however, has change substantially since the first addition of this book. More recently, experts recommend only a few days of physical rest followed by gradual resumption of nonrisk, noncontact physical activity below the level at which symptoms are exacerbated.

Complete physical rest until full resolution of symptoms was recommended in the summary and agreement statement from the first international consensus on concussion in sport. This recommendation was further emphasized and discussed in the subsequent statements from that meeting, which is held every four years or so. In addition the concept of cognitive rest was introduced at the summary and agreement statement from the second international consensus on concussion in sports. At this time it was recommended that athletes who are still symptomatic from a concussion avoid activities that demand concentration and attention including participation in school.

Although I was not present at the initial international consensus meetings, I do not believe that the participants thought that the recommendation for rest would be employed so strictly by treating clinicians. Indeed, stories of "cocoon" therapy have emerged where athletes have been instructed to lay down for most of the day in a quiet dark room without engaging in any activity in an effort to try and speed the recovery from concussion. As noted, there have been several studies published in the last few years that suggest this type of restriction of physical activity may be unnecessary and, in fact, may be detrimental to recovery from concussion. Instead, it may be associated with symptoms of its own that are often mistaken for symptoms of a concussion.

In a study of 95 student athletes cared for at the University of Pittsburgh Medical Center, the amount of activity athletes engaged in while recovering from a concussion was measured. The level of activity student athletes engaged in during recovery was compared to their symptom level and performance on computerized neurocognitive assessments. Those athletes engaging in a moderate level of physical activity performed best, while athletes engaging in both a high level and low level of physical activity performed worse. The authors concluded that perhaps engaging in some physical activity was beneficial in the recovery from sport-related concussion.

In an additional study conducted at Boston Children's Hospital, the physical activity of athletes recovering from a sport-related concussion was monitored between visits and compared to the overall duration of concussion symptoms. Increased levels of physical activity were not associated with a prolonged recovery. In fact, among adolescent athletes, higher levels of physical activity were associated with a shorter duration of symptoms.

Perhaps most convincingly, 88 adolescent patients managed at the Medical College of Wisconsin were randomly placed in two groups. One of the groups was given a recommendation for strict rest. The other group was given a recommendation for a few days of rest followed by gradual, stepwise return to activity. The group that was given a recommendation for strict rest reported more severe symptoms and took longer to recover than the group that gradually returned to activity after a few days of rest.

As a result of these and other studies, the recommendations for physical rest after a sport-related concussion have changed. In the most recent consensus statement from the International Conference on Concussion in Sports the recommendation has been made for a brief period of rest, 24 to 48 hours after injury, after which time patients can become gradually more active while staying below the level at which their symptoms are exacerbated. Still, athletes are recommended to avoid contact or other activities with an increased risk of trauma to the head until they are at least completely symptom-free and cleared to participate in those activities by a clinician experienced in the management of sport-related concussion.

Most athletes enjoy exercise. It improves their mood, their health, their self-image. In such athletes, a prolonged absence from physical activity can lead to depression and irritability. While the occurrence of this will hopefully decrease given the new recommendations that allow for some physical activity shortly after injury, many athletes still may experience some mood changes as a result of not being able to fully participate in their sports. When this occurs, counseling with a sports psychologist is often effective. Through counseling, these symptoms can be alleviated; and athletes can learn coping strategies to help them deal with their injuries. Occasionally, medications can be considered.

In addition to early physical rest, increasing the amount of time they sleep may help athletes who sustain a sport-related concussion recover faster. If an athlete typically sleeps 8½ hours per night, increasing to 10 or more hours a night may help with recovery. Some athletes find sleeping for such a long period difficult. In those cases, taking a nap during the day may help the athlete get some extra sleep during his or her recovery. Unfortunately, insomnia, which is an inability to obtain adequate sleep, is a common symptom of concussion. Thus, while increased amounts of sleep may assist with recovery, they can be hard to obtain. Some strategies for addressing insomnia are discussed later. Again, it is hoped that with the new recommendations that allow for increased physical activity shortly after injury, the effects on overall daytime energy and sleep disturbance will be minimized thereby negating the need for many of these strategies.

Not all concussions are the same. Similarly, the recovery from concussion is not always the same. Therefore, the management of concussion including the amount of physical activity recommended varies and should be discussed with the clinician managing the injury.

COGNITIVE REST

As discussed in the previous chapter, cognitive activities, those that require thinking, remembering, concentrating, or reasoning, should be avoided during the first few days of recovery from a concussion. This will often necessitate an absence from school. Usually, this can be accomplished without too much trouble for the first few days after injury. Some athletes, however, will have symptoms that last longer than the first week after their injury. For these athletes, the recommendations have again changed since the first addition of this book, allowing for more cognitive activity even prior to full symptom resolution often with the implementation of academic accommodations, which are discussed further later. Similar to physical activity, studies of cognitive activity after injury have suggested that allowing some activity may improve outcomes. Several of the studies mentioned earlier were not limited only to physical activity but also allowed for an increase in cognitive activity that likely contributed to the improvement and outcomes. In addition, a study of 335 athletes cared for at Boston Children's Hospital monitored the cognitive activity of patients recovering from a sport-related concussion. They noticed that those athletes engaging in the highest levels of cognitive activity had the longest recoveries. They also noted, however, that those athletes engaging in minimal, mild, and moderate amounts of cognitive activity all recovered at approximately the same rate. The findings suggest that while some mild restrictions in cognitive activity may be useful during recovery from concussion, more moderate levels of cognitive activity do not appear to be harmful. Combining these findings with those of other studies discussed earlier, it is likely that allowing some cognitive activity during recovery from concussion after a brief period of rest is likely helpful.

In addition, there are several other reasons for avoiding absences from school. Athletes learn more in school than simply the subjects in which they are enrolled. They learn to make friends, respect authority, manage a schedule, interact with their peers, and socialize. As discussed earlier, the social isolation from being restricted from school attendance can result in symptoms of its own including depression, low energy, and overall irritability. Much of this is learned through less formal means than classroom teaching itself. Furthermore, although many young athletes do not readily admit it, school is fun. This is where they see their friends and where most of their social interactions take place. Learning social skills is essential. In fact, I would argue that learning social skills is ultimately more important in life than learning the classroom subjects. Don't get me wrong, learning mathematics, reading, writing, English grammar, science, and other core subjects is extremely important. But you can be the most knowledgeable person in the world, and if you have poor social skills, no one will want to work with you. You will find it hard to get a job, and even harder to be successful at one. Those who learn to treat others with respect, to interact with teammates and classmates, to respect authority, and to stand up for themselves while still being agreeable, are more pleasant to work with. Thus, they often have an easier time finding a job, and being successful at a given job.

Reentering into school while still recovering from a concussion, however, is not an easy task. Schoolwork and homework require the very same activities that make symptoms worse: remembering, reasoning, concentrating, and thinking.

Table 8.1
Graduated Return-to-School Strategy

Stage	Aim	Activity	Goal of Each Step
1	Daily activities at home that do not give the child symptoms	Typical activities of the child during the day as long as they do not increase symptoms (e.g., reading, texting, screen time). Start with 5–15 minutes at a time and gradually build up	Gradual return to typical activities
2	School activities	Homework, reading or other cognitive activities outside of the classroom	Increased tolerance to cognitive work
3	Return to school part-time	Gradual introduction of schoolwork. It may need to start with a partial school day or at increased breaks during the day	Increase academic activities
4	Return to school full time	Gradually progressed school activities until a full day can be tolerated	Return to full academic activities and catch up on missed work

Source: Adapted from McCrory, P., W. Meeuwisse, and J. Dvorak, et al. "Consensus statement on concussion in sport: The Fifth International Conference on Concussion in Sport held in Berlin, October 2016." *Br J Sports Med*. Published Online First: April 26, 2017. doi: 10.1136/bjsports-2017-097699.

Furthermore, the concussed brain is not functioning properly. The speed with which a concussed athlete is able to process information is reduced. The ability to concentrate is decreased. Reaction time is slowed. Memory is poor. Therefore, concussed athletes often have difficulties in school and significant decreases in their grades. In recognition of this problem, the consensus statement on concussion in sports from the Fifth International Conference on Concussion in Sport held in Berlin in October 2016 includes a segment on returning to school as well as a graduated return to school strategy that includes a table of stages through which the student athlete should progress (Table 8.1).

In order to help athletes stay in school, keep up with their course work, and minimize any negative impacts their concussion might otherwise have on their grades, concussed athletes are entitled to academic accommodations. These should be put in place as soon as it becomes clear the athlete will not recover quickly. Academic accommodations are exceptions to the normal school rules and timetables that allow concussed athletes to reenter school prior to complete recovery. Some of the more commonly used accommodations are:

1. Giving concussed students preprinted class notes, so they can listen to the teacher during class, as opposed to concentrating on both listening to the teacher and copying down all of the information for later reference.

2. Giving concussed athletes extra time on tests and quizzes. Since the speed with which concussed athletes are able to process information has been slowed, and the memory of concussed athletes is temporarily diminished, it takes longer to complete tasks that they were able to complete rather quickly prior to the injury. Thus, extra time is required to take tests and quizzes during recovery.

3. Offering concussed athletes tutors to help them with their homework. Many students who have not sustained a concussion take advantage of tutoring. During recovery from a concussion, tutoring may be helpful.

4. Allowing the athlete to go to the nurse's office to lie down if concussion symptoms increase during the school day. Even with academic accommodations in place, school attendance can exacerbate symptoms. Rest will help relieve them.

5. Reducing the athlete's work load. Although teachers hate when I say this, some homework assignments are more important than others. Many readers will recall having to memorize the capitols of the 50 states at some point in their academic careers. While I do believe there is some value in this, it is far more important to learn arithmetic. Therefore, athletes recovering from a concussion should not be required to complete such assignments as "memorize the capitols of the 50 states," but rather, should focus their efforts on learning mathematics, science and other such material.

6. Offering concussed athletes extensions on their homework assignments. As we have discussed, athletes recovering from a concussion will often need more time to accomplish tasks that once came to them quite readily. Similarly, they will need to take breaks when their symptoms increase. This prolongs the time needed to complete assignments. Thus, extensions on these assignments allow the athletes to complete them properly, and to the best of their capabilities.

7. Some athletes will need to limit their course load. Rather than taking 6–7 courses at a time, some athletes might only be able to manage 2–4 courses at a time. They might only attend a half day of school as opposed to a whole day. When this is necessary, I recommend athletes maintain courses that build upon themselves, such as mathematics and science. You cannot learn how to multiply two numbers each containing multiple digits, unless you first learned to multiply two single integers together. Mathematics generally builds on itself in this way. It can be difficult to return to math class in March if you missed the material covered in February. Classes like English and history tend to be somewhat more forgiving. You can read Oliver Twist, even if you have never read Animal Farm. The two have little to do with each other.

There are several other strategies that may help athletes accomplish their school work while recovering from a sport-related concussion. Many healthy, uninjured students will complete their homework for the day in one session. They will sit down at a desk or table for several hours straight and complete all of their assignments. While this is a perfectly reasonable way of doing it when healthy, such a long period of concentration, thinking and reasoning will often exacerbate a concussed athlete's symptoms. A better approach during recovery is to accomplish homework assignments in small chunks of time. Doing one's homework in 20 minute intervals with 5–10 minute breaks in between may help prevent symptoms from worsening.

A few things should be remembered about academic accommodations. First, they are temporary. When an athlete has recovered, there is no longer a need for academic accommodations. They should then be discontinued. Second, academic accommodations are a two edged sword. While they may seem advantageous to some readers, most athletes dislike them. The athlete is still responsible for the work covered in class. Academic accommodations allow for the forgiveness of some minor assignments, and allow the athlete to postpone more important assignments. But tests, quizzes and more major assignments need to be made up. And no athlete likes the thought of making up weeks' worth of quizzes, tests, and homework assignments once they have recovered from their concussion. Furthermore, it can be hard to advance in school without the proper background. Therefore, even if work is forgiven, if the student athlete does not learn the material that was covered in their absence, it may be difficult to learn future material.

Ultimately, the goal of academic accommodations is to allow concussed students to stay in school and keep up with their school work as best as they can without 1) making their symptoms worse, 2) delaying their recovery more than necessary, and 3) allowing their grades to decline unnecessarily.

Prolonged recovery from sport-related concussion: For many if not most cases of prolonged recovery from a sport-related concussion, it is unclear whether or not the symptoms are attributable to a concussion from which athletes are incompletely recovered or rather, attributable to other potential causes. The symptoms of concussion are nonspecific, as was discussed previously in Chapter 7. That is to say, the symptoms of concussion can also be caused by many other conditions including dehydration, depression, hangover, viral illness, among others. In fact, since the first addition of this book was published, there have been studies that suggest prolonged restrictions on activities that were used by well-intentioned clinicians who recommended strict physical and cognitive rest, may have resulted in symptoms similar to those caused by concussion. While the actual cellular changes of concussion recovered, these symptoms induced by the restriction on activities may have led to athletes and their clinicians believing that the concussion was not yet recovered. This may have led to unnecessary restrictions in activities and the misbelief that these concussions resulted in prolonged recoveries.

In a summary of the existing literature on physical and cognitive rest and restriction in activities often recommended in the setting of sport-related concussion, Difazio and colleagues describe several possible harms. One possible harm is what's known as the nocebo effect. Most readers will be familiar with what is known as the placebo effect, whereby an inert substance, such as saline or a sugar pill, results in a beneficial effect on the patient's condition if the patient is first led to believe that such a beneficial effect will occur. There is also a lesser known phenomenon known as the nocebo effect, whereby the belief that one is sick leads to a decrease in one's condition and feelings of sickness, perhaps attributable, in part, to hyperawareness of potential symptoms or signs of illness. A second possible harm noted by Difazio and his colleagues is psychological effects of restrictions on activities. One can imagine that social isolation due to recommended restrictions in both cognitive and physical activity can lead to depression. Furthermore, for student athletes there can be a substantial amount of emotional stress associated with falling behind in school. It can be daunting to have to make up multiple days' or weeks' worth of assignments, tests, and quizzes in multiple subjects after missing school due to "cognitive rest" while recovering from a concussion. This emotional stress can lead to symptoms of its own, including difficulty sleeping, which is associated with symptoms that can often be mistaken for symptoms of concussion, such as low energy, difficulty concentrating, and headaches, among others. Finally, this can be compounded with the third potential harm noted by Difazio and colleagues, physical deconditioning. For an athlete who is used to regular exercise, the lack of such exercise can lead to symptoms of its own. They are no longer burning a substantial amount of energy during the day, thus leading to difficulty with sleep. This can lead to decreased daytime energy, difficulty with concentration, headaches, and poor mental focus. Physical deconditioning itself can lead to decreased energy as it is well-established that regular exercise leads to increased daytime alertness. Putting all of the findings of previous literature together, these authors argue quite convincingly that overly strict restrictions in activities in an attempt to facilitate recovery from concussion likely lead to symptoms that are mistakenly attributed to incomplete recovery from concussion and the misbelief that a concussion recovery has been prolonged.

In addition, animal models of concussion and other forms of traumatic brain injury have suggested that blood flow to the brain is decreased after injury for a period of days to weeks. More recently, studies of patients who have sustained concussions, including sport-related concussions, have shown changes in blood flow to the brain, as well as the regulation of blood flow to the brain, after injury. Investigators from Cincinnati Children's Medical Center used magnetic resonance imaging (MRI) to show changes in blood flow to the brain among pediatric patients who had sustained a sport-related concussion that lasted even beyond a month after injury.

In a thorough review of the literature on this topic, investigators from Spaulding Rehabilitation Hospital have suggested a possible hypothesis connecting changes in the regulation of blood flow to the brain and the symptoms often attributed to concussion. Evidence suggests that a concussion to lead to a disruption of the regulation of blood flow to the brain. Symptoms similar to those that are associated with concussion, such as dizziness, low energy, difficulty with concentration and memory, among others, can develop as a result of disruption of the normal regulation of blood flow to the brain. Regular exercise is associated with better regulation of blood flow to the brain and the abrupt cessation of exercise in someone who is used to regularly exercising can lead to worsening regulation of blood flow to the brain. Therefore, it could be that athletes who are used to regular exercise sustain a concussion and that this leads to classic concussion symptoms such as difficulty with memory and concentration, headaches, dizziness, among others. They are then instructed to stop exercising and this abrupt cessation of regular exercise leads to a disruption in the regulation of blood flow to the brain. This disruption of blood flow leads, itself, to symptoms such as headaches, dizziness, difficulty with concentration and memory that mimic concussion symptoms. While their concussion fully resolves, the symptoms brought on by the disruption of regulation of blood flow to the brain persist and are mistakenly attributed to a concussion from which they are believed to be incompletely recovered. In some cases this may have led to clinicians recommending more strict restrictions on exercise, thereby exacerbating the problem. This hypothesis is further supported by the observation that introducing some light aerobic exercise to those in recovery from concussion can reverse symptoms and shorten the duration of symptoms. In a series of studies conducted at the State University of New York at Buffalo, Dr. John Leddy and colleagues have shown that exercise implemented during recovery from concussion is safe, likely reduces symptom level and the duration of symptoms, and helps restore the regulation of blood flow to the brain.

For these reasons, it seems the best approach to concussion management involves a few days of rest, both physical and cognitive, followed by gradual return to cognitive activity and non-risk, noncontact physical activity, even if symptoms have not fully abated after the first few days of rest. Common sense would dictate that activities that result in a substantial increase in the patient's symptoms continue to be avoided and replaced with activities of a more moderate level of intensity. Certainly, activities that place the athlete at risk for additional trauma to the head should be avoided until full symptom resolution, full re-achievement of any available baseline data, and official medical clearance by a clinician experienced in the assessment and management of sport-related concussion.

In fact, the consensus statement from the Fifth International Conference on Concussion in Sports was held in October 2016 states, "after a brief period of rest during the acute phase (24–48 hours) after injury, patients can be encouraged to become gradually and progressively more active while staying below their cognitive and physical symptom–exacerbation thresholds (i.e., activity level should not bring on or worsen their symptoms)."

OTHER POTENTIAL THERAPIES

If you or your athlete is taking a long time to recover from a concussion or experiencing persistent symptoms after a concussion regardless of the ultimate cause of the symptoms, consider seeing a specialist in the assessment and management of sport-related concussion. Although there is no medicine that has been shown to effectively speed the recovery form a concussive brain injury, many of the symptoms can be treated medically. Most physicians will be unfamiliar with these treatments. Many are still being developed, and therefore, will be unknown to many clinicians. Seeing someone who specializes in the assessment and management of concussion may open up other possibilities for treatment. Some specific symptoms are discussed here.

Headache

Headache is the most common symptom of concussion in general and of sport-related concussion specifically. Often, headaches will resolve within the first few days to weeks after a sport-related concussion with only physical and cognitive rest. But for some athletes, headaches will persist. Ironically, those who seem, at first, to have sustained only a minor injury, often suffer worse headaches afterwards, and suffer headaches for a longer period of time, than those who initially seemed to have a more severe injury.

For the first few days after injury, obtaining physical and cognitive rest will help alleviate headaches caused by concussion. Similarly, avoiding prolonged periods of concentration, thinking and reasoning can help prevent headaches during the first few days after recovery. Even later on in recovery, prolonged cognitive exertion or prolonged physical exertion makes exacerbate symptoms. Therefore, much like the recommendations mentioned earlier for athletes in school, all athletes should try to break up cognitive tasks that they cannot avoid into many small chunks of time, as opposed to focusing on a given cognitive task for one long stretch of time. Exercise should be limited to non-risk, noncontact aerobic in resistance training that does not exacerbate symptoms.

In response to these post-concussive headaches, many athletes will start taking common over the counter medications such as acetaminophen, ibuprofen and aspirin. Certainly, these medications are useful for treating headaches in general. They are safe and well tolerated by most patients. However, they should not be taken routinely to treat the headaches of a sport-related concussion. They tend to be ineffective in treating post-concussive headaches. Oftentimes, athletes take these medications three or four times per day in an attempt to alleviate the headaches. Once an athlete has been taking these medications multiple times per day for several days or weeks, it can be hard to stop them. Any attempt to stop the medications will result in "rebound headaches." Rebound headaches are similar to withdrawal headaches. Many readers who enjoy coffee, tea, and other caffeinated beverages will be familiar with withdrawal headaches. Those who enjoy these drinks daily will often experience withdrawal headaches when they go a day without caffeine. Similarly, when concussed athletes taking acetaminophen, ibuprofen or aspirin regularly for headaches try to stop the medications, they will experience a rebound headache. Athletes will often mistake these rebound headaches for persistent post-concussive headaches. This makes it difficult to determine when the athlete has recovered. Therefore, for the first few days to weeks after injury, I recommend athletes respond to the headaches by trying to obtain more rest, and by limiting their activities. Other medications are more effective for treating post-concussive headaches that do not resolve over the first few days to weeks, and therefore, become a significant, daily problem.

If headaches persist, and are negatively impacting an athlete's quality of life, there are multiple other strategies and medications that can be used to treat the headaches of a concussion. Oftentimes, at the Sports Concussion Clinic at Children's Hospital Boston, we will offer the athlete a preventative headache medication. One such medication is called amitriptyline. Amitriptyline is most commonly used as an antidepressant, medication given to patients who suffer from clinical depression. However, it is also effective at treating headaches: migraine headaches, tension headaches, cluster headaches, and post-concussive headaches. It has been studied specifically in patients who have headaches after sustaining a concussion. It decreases the frequency with which patients recovering from a concussion suffer headaches. It reduces the intensity of headaches, when they do occur, in patients recovering from a concussion. In fact, amitriptyline is so useful in treating post-concussive headaches that often a dose as small as 1/10th of the dose used to treat depression is effective in reducing the intensity and frequency of post-concussive headaches. At such a small dosages, amitriptyline tends to be well tolerated by patients. Side effects tend to be minimal. However, sleepiness is one side effect that is common, even at the small dosages used to treat post-concussive headaches. As many patients suffering from post-concussive headaches also have insomnia, this side effect can be advantageous. Amitriptyline can be used to treat both the headaches and the insomnia. There has been a recent study that suggested that perhaps the use of amitriptyline to treat headaches is no better than placebo. These headaches were not headaches secondary to a concussion specifically, however. Many treating clinicians still use this medication given the fact that it is safe and some patients seem to benefit from it. Either way, when deciding to take medication it is best to discuss the risks and benefits with your treating clinician.

Although it is common to use the amitriptyline to treat post concussive headaches, especially in younger athletes, there are many other potential therapies and medications that can be used to treat post-concussive headaches. Therapies such as biofeedback, psychotherapy, physical therapy, and trigger point injections can be used to treat post-concussive headaches, either by themselves or in conjunction with medications. Other medications that physicians may consider for the treatment of post-concussive headaches include beta-blockers, calcium channel blockers, valproic acid, triptans, topiramate, gabapentin, pregabalin, and dihydroergotamine. If you or your athlete has persistent headaches that negatively impact the quality of life for weeks after sustaining a sport-related concussion, you should discuss the best potential therapies for treating those headaches with the physician managing your sport-related concussion. Many times, prior to starting such medications, physicians will order further tests to assess for other potential injuries as well as the general health of the patient. This should not alarm you. Although it is not always necessary, these tests are commonly performed prior to starting new medications.

If the first one or two medications recommended fails to significantly alleviate the athlete's headaches, consultation with a headache specialist can sometimes be useful. Headache specialists are most often are neurologists. At the Sports Concussion Clinic at Children's Hospital Boston, we work closely with several neurologists who have significant experience and expertise in treating headaches. I often refer athletes to these neurologists if I am unable to control their headaches with the first one or two medications tried.

Insomnia

Insomnia is the ability to obtain adequate sleep. As it is common, many readers will have heard of insomnia or even experienced insomnia at some point in their lives. Insomnia is one of the most common symptoms of concussion, especially in athletes who do not recover quickly. There are several strategies for helping an athlete who is suffering from insomnia after a concussion to get some sleep.

The first and easiest strategy is to rid the athlete's bedroom of all potentially distracting items. Today's athletes are surrounded by distractions. Their bedrooms are often filled with electronics such as stereos, videogames, televisions, cell phones, laptop computers, iPods, and more. They are constantly bombarded with social messages through phone calls, text-messages, instant messages, emails, Facebook messages, My Space messages, etc. Eliminating such distractions from the bedroom and having the athlete lie down in a quiet, dark room will help induce sleep. Simply turning these gadgets off or switching them to vibrate is less effective. The mere presence of these devices can be distracting. Not only electronics should be removed. The presences of even a "to do" list, schedule, or daily planner can bring to mind all the tasks that lay ahead. This can cause stress and anxiety, which prevent sleep.

Similarly, concussed athletes suffering from insomnia should avoid potential stimulants such as caffeine or nicotine. Alcohol may also cause difficulties sleeping. For this, as well as other reasons, an athlete recovering from a concussion should avoid alcohol.

If these interventions do not result in adequate sleep there are medications that may be considered. As with all medications, these should be discussed with and supervised by a physician.

A safe and common medication often used to treat insomnia is called melatonin. Melatonin is actually not a medication; it is a hormone. All of us have melatonin in our blood. It is secreted into the blood by a gland in the brain known as the pineal gland. When it gets dark and the temperature drops, the pineal gland secretes melatonin into the blood stream. Melatonin makes us feel sleepy. This is why we get tired when it is dark, especially if it the temperature has cooled. Taking melatonin by mouth can help athletes suffering from insomnia after a concussion fall asleep.

As noted earlier, amitriptyline can be used to treat post-concussive insomnia, especially in athletes who are also suffering from post-concussive headaches. In addition, many other therapies and medications can be used to treat insomnia. Non-medical therapies such as chronotherapy, psychotherapy, herbal teas, relaxation techniques, and phototherapy may be useful. Medications such as trazodone, zolpidem, other tricyclic antidepressants (besides amitriptyline), and various other medications may be helpful in certain situations, but these decisions are best left to providers with substantial experience in managing insomnia in the setting of sport-related concussion. As always, it is best to discuss the options that are best for you or your athlete with an expert in the assessment and management of sport-related concussion. Lastly, it is hoped that with the new recommendations to allow resumption of physical activity shortly after injury sleep disturbance will be minimized.

Depression

Depression is common in athletes who do not recover quickly from their concussions. The most important thing you can do if you are having depression after a concussion is tell someone such as a doctor, a school nurse, a counselor, a psychologist or another professional who can get you help. This is especially true for athletes who feel hopeless. Thoughts of harming oneself or killing oneself are particularly concerning and should be reported immediately. Fortunately, such profound depression is rare. More commonly, athletes are simply saddened by their injury, by the fact that they cannot participate fully in sports, and by the fact that they have more difficulty with schoolwork and other cognitive tasks. It is frustrating. Depression is understandable. But it can usually be overcome with proper treatment.

Seeing a sports psychologist can be helpful in treating depression after a sport-related concussion. Sports psychologists are trained in psychology, and have extra training in the psychological issues specifically related to sports and athletes. In addition to improving the athlete's mood and treating the depression, a sports psychologist can teach the athlete coping strategies, ways of dealing with their injury, with their cognitive dysfunction, and with the limitations imposed on their activities and functioning as a result of their concussion.

In certain circumstances, allowing athletes to return to aerobic exercise is safe. This can go a long way in improving an athlete's mood and overall disposition. This option should be discussed with the clinician managing the athlete's concussion.

Finally, sometimes these interventions are not enough, and the athlete remains depressed despite them. In such cases, medication may be considered. This option should be discussed with the athlete's doctor. Many doctors will refer an athlete to another clinician who is experienced in treating depression with medicine, as opposed to prescribing it themselves.

Cognitive Dysfunction

As noted previously, cognitive processes are those that involve thinking, reasoning, concentrating and remembering. These processes are negatively impacted by concussion. Thinking becomes slower. Memory becomes worse. Concentration becomes difficult. This can be frustrating, especially for student athletes. As with all the signs and symptoms of concussion, these problems should resolve shortly, over the course of a few days to weeks. In some small percentage of athletes, however, these problems persist for weeks to months. Many athletes seek treatment for these problems. The best and most effective treatments are discussed in the section on cognitive rest and academic accommodations. However, some athletes' problems will be so severe and last for so long, that they negatively impact the athlete's quality of life to such an extent that the athlete seeks other treatments.

Unfortunately, there is no proven, generally accepted therapy for treating the cognitive dysfunction caused by sport-related concussion or concussive brain injuries sustained outside of sports. There are, however, some potential medications that might be considered. Some medical studies have shown that these medications can help maintain the brain function of people who have sustained a traumatic brain injury. Other studies have shown no benefit. These medications act directly on the cells of the brain, known as neurons. Like all medications, there are side effects associated with them. Athletes taking them should be monitored closely. Before deciding whether or not an athlete will take one of these medications, the athlete should understand all of the potential risks and the likelihood of benefit. These medications should only be prescribed by a physician with expertise and experience in the assessment and management of concussive brain injuries.

Although more common in more severe forms of traumatic brain injury, cognitive rehabilitation is another potential therapy for the treatment of sport-related concussions. The Brain Injury Association of America defines cognitive rehabilitation as "a systematically applied set of medical and therapeutic services designed to improve cognitive functioning and participation in activities that may be affected by difficulties in one or more cognitive domains." Simply, it is a way of retraining the brain to perform activities that, prior to injury, it was able to perform readily. There is little evidence supporting its use after sport-related concussions. Since most athletes will recover from sport-related concussions relatively quickly, the routine use of cognitive rehabilitation after sport-related concussion is unnecessary. However, for athletes suffering from prolonged cognitive dysfunction after sustaining a sport-related concussion, cognitive rehabilitation may be considered.

Vestibular and Oculomotor Dysfunction

After sustaining a sport-related concussion, some athletes will suffer vestibular problems. The vestibular system consists of parts of the brain and the inner ear that help control balance, coordination, and eye movements. This dysfunction may arise from the concussion itself or from concomitant injuries that occurred to the inner ear at the same time as concussion. Oculomotor dysfunction may be related to a disruption of the vestibular system or maybe an independent and distinct set of problems. Either way, there is some preliminary evidence that suggests that both vestibular dysfunction after concussion and oculomotor dysfunction after concussion might benefit from guided vestibular and oculomotor therapy. For athletes whose symptoms persist more than a few weeks after concussion and are associated with difficulties with balance, dizziness, or vision problems, referral to a vestibular therapist, optometrist, or other appropriate specialist might be considered.

In summary, the vast majority of athletes will recover from a sport-related concussion quickly, within days to weeks. A brief period of relative physical and cognitive rest will often be the only therapies necessary to achieve a complete recovery from a sport-related concussion. Most of the other therapies discussed in this chapter will be unnecessary for most readers and their athletes. However, a small percentage of concussed athletes will suffer prolonged symptoms, lasting weeks to months. Some athletes will have such profound symptoms, that their quality of life will be negatively impacted by their injuries. For this small minority, other therapies should be considered to assist them with their recovery. The potential risks and adverse effects of these medications must be considered and weighed against the likelihood of benefit. These therapies should be tailored to address the athletes' most bothersome symptoms. Athletes engaging in these potential therapies should be closely monitored in conjunction with a clinician experienced in the assessment and management of sport-related concussions or concussive brain injuries in general.

SUGGESTED READINGS

Beers, S. R., A. Skold, C. E. Dixon, and P. D. Adelson. Neurobehavioral effects of amantadine after pediatric traumatic brain injury: A preliminary report. *J Head Trauma Rehabil*, 2005, 20: 450–463.

Brown, N. J., R. C. Mannix, M. J. O'Brien, D. Gostine, M. W. Collins, W. P. Meehan III. Effect of cognitive activity level on duration of post-concussion symptoms. *Pediatrics*, 2014, 133(2): e299–e304.

Chew, E., and R. D. Zafonte. Pharmacological management of neurobehavioral disorders following traumatic brain injury—A state-of-the-art review. *J Rehabil Res Dev*, 2009, 46(6): 851–879.

Corwin, D. J., et al. Vestibular deficits following use concussion. *J Pediatr*, 2015, 166(5): 1221–1225.

Howell, D. R., R. C. Mannix, B. Quinn, J. A. Taylor, C. O. Tan, W. P. Meehan III. Physical activity level and symptom duration are not associated after concussion. *Am J Sport Med*, 2016, 44(4): 1040–1046.

Leddy, J. J., J. L. Cox, J. G. Baker, D. S. Wack, D. R. Pendergast, R. Zivadinov, and B. Willer. Exercise treatment for postconcussion syndrome: A pilot study of changes in functional magnetic resonance imaging activation, physiology, and symptoms. *J Head Trauma Rehabil*, 2013, 28(4): 241–249.

Lenaerts, M. E., and J. R. Couch. Posttraumatic headache. *Curr Treat Options Neurol*, 2004, 6: 507–517.

Master, C. L., et al. Vision diagnoses are common after concussion in adolescents. *Clin Pediatr (Phila)*, 2016, 55(3): 260–267.

Maugans, T. A., C. Farley, M. Altaye, J. Leach, and K. M. Cecil. Pediatric sports-related concussion produces cerebral blood flow alterations. *Pediatrics*, 2012, 129(1): 28–37.

McCrory, P., et al. Consensus statement on concussion in sport: The Fifth International Conference on Concussion in Sport held in Berlin, October 2016. *Br J Sports Med*, 2017 [Epub ahead of print].

McCrory, P., et al. Consensus statement on concussion in sport: The 3rd International Conference on Concussion in Sport held in Zurich, November 2008. *J Athl Train*, 2009, 44(4): 434–448.

Meehan, W. P., III, P. d'Hemecourt, and R. D. Comstock. High school concussions in the 2008–2009 academic year: Mechanism, symptoms, and management. *Am J Sports Med*, 2010, 38(12): 2405–2409.

Moore, B. M., et al. Outcomes following a vestibular rehabilitation and aerobic training program to address persistent postconcussion symptoms. *J Allied Health*, 2016, 45(4): e59–e68.

Rao, V., and P. Rollings. Sleep disturbances following traumatic brain injury. *Curr Treat Options Neurol*, 2002, 4: 77–87.

Storey, E. P., et al. Near point of convergence after concussion in children. *Optom Vis Sci.*, 2017, 94(1): 96–100.

Tan, C. O., W. P. Meehan III, G. L. Iverson, and J. A. Taylor. Cerebrovascular regulation, exercise, and mild traumatic brain injury. *Neurology*, 2014, 83(18): 1665–1672.

Tenovuo, O. Pharmacological enhancement of cognitive and behavioral deficits after traumatic brain injury. *Curr Opin Neurol*, 2006, 19: 528–533.

Whyte, J., T. Hart, K. Schuster, M. Fleming, M. Polansky, and H. B. Coslett. Effects of methylphenidate on attentional function after traumatic brain injury. A randomized, placebo-controlled trial. *Am J Phys Med Rehabil*, 1997, 76: 440–450.

9

ASSESSING RECOVERY FROM CONCUSSION: WHEN IS IT SAFE FOR AN ATHLETE TO RETURN TO SPORTS?

On Sunday September 12, 2010, the Philadelphia Eagles were playing the Green Bay packers. It was the second quarter. While tackling Green Bay's wide receiver, Greg Jennings, the head of Eagles' linebacker Stewart Bradley bounced off of the right hip of his teammate and fellow linebacker Ernie Sims. On video replay, Stewart's head was seen snapping sharply back while twisting to his right. When the play was over, Bradley struggled to stand up. After approximately seven seconds of balancing himself tenuously on all four limbs, he rose to his feet. He stumbled forward, only to fall again, face first, onto the ground. He was dazed, stunned, off-balance. His fellow players knew something was wrong. Even his opponent, Green Bay's Greg Jennings, started waving the medical staff onto the field to tend to Bradley.

Stewart Bradley was concussed.

Yet later in that same quarter, Bradley was returned to play. This sparked a lot of controversy in the sports community, with sports writers and sports blog enthusiasts taking Philadelphia coach Andy Reid, and the Eagles' medical staff to task. According to the guidelines adopted by the National Football League less than a year earlier, a player who suffers a concussion should not return to play on the same day. The Eagles responded by saying Bradley had been able to "go through the protocol." But with the nation watching on television, it seemed that Bradley, who had clearly suffered a concussion, was returned to play during the same game.

This chapter will discuss the strategies used for monitoring an athlete's recovery over time. Concussion monitoring focuses on three main categories: (1) the recovery from symptoms, (2) the recovery of brain function and (3) the recovery of balance and other motor tasks. The determination of recovery is made by assessing these three indicators of injury. Often, after an athlete is believed to have fully recovered, an additional rest period is recommended. When an athlete is cleared to return to play, there are international guidelines through which athletes should progress, prior to participating in competition.

Ideally, there will be a baseline value for each of the three main components of recovery (symptoms, balance, and cognitive function).

Athletes will be monitored until they return to their baseline scores. If no baseline data are available for a given athlete, then clinicians will do their best to determine when complete recovery has occurred. Often, in the absence of baseline data, longer symptom-free waiting period will be added to the recovery, prior to clearing an athlete for contact. This extra rest period will often be longer for younger athletes. Prior to clearing an athlete to resume contact or collision play, baseline data should be collected so they may be used in the unfortunate event of future concussions.

SYMPTOMS

As noted previously, symptoms are most often measured using a symptom inventory. An example of a commonly used symptom inventory is shown in Figure 7.1. Most athletes are given a list of symptoms, followed by a scale of severity from 0 to 6, where 0 means the athlete is not experiencing the symptom, and 6 means the symptom is as severe as the athlete can imagine. The athlete is asked to circle the number that corresponds to the degree of severity for each of the symptoms listed. These numbers can then be added together in order to get a total post-concussion symptom scale score. For example, if an athlete has a pretty bad headache, some nausea, some trouble falling asleep, and decreased energy on the day he fills out the symptom inventory, his scale might look like this:

Figure 9.1
Example of Part of a Post-concussion Symptom Scale

Headache	0	1	2	3	4	5	6
Nausea	0	1	2	3	4	5	6
Difficulty sleeping	0	1	2	3	4	5	6
Decreased energy	0	1	2	3	4	5	6

If he is not experiencing any other symptoms, a "0" would be circled for the remainder of the symptoms included in the inventory.

5 for headache + 2 for nausea + 1 for difficulty sleeping + 3 for decreased energy = 11.

Thus, his total symptom score would be 11.

Many people will have some mild symptoms even when they are not injured. Some people have headaches and nausea from time to time. Some have difficulty falling asleep even when they are not injured or concussed. By measuring these symptoms before a concussion, clinicians can determine whether an athlete's symptoms are worse after their injury. Similarly, they can see how long it takes for athletes symptoms to return to their preseason, "baseline" level. By measuring all symptoms before the start of the season, athletes who were having some symptoms before their concussion won't mistakenly be considered concussed after they have recovered, even if they are still experiencing the same headaches, nausea, decreased energy and difficulty sleeping they were having before their injury. For athletes who have no symptoms when they are in their usual state of health, their initial, preseason, baseline symptoms inventory score will be 0.

One can imagine, however, some athletes will show up for their preseason assessment after they were up late at night studying. Or, on the day of their preseason baseline measurement, they might have a cold or the flu. Thus, they may have many symptoms when they complete their "baseline" symptom inventory, which are not "baseline" at all. They are due to the fact that the athlete just happens to be tired or ill on the day the inventory is taken. Thus, another approach is to only measure those symptoms that are due to a concussion. When performed this way, every athlete should score a 0 at the start of the season (unless they are recovering from a concussion from a prior season). When the baseline symptom inventory is completed in this way, athletes who sustain a concussion should be asked to complete follow-up symptom inventories after injury by circling *only those symptoms that started at the time of their concussion and have not yet gone away.*

Both approaches to symptom inventories are reasonable. Whichever method is used, no athlete should be returned to play until the symptoms due to his or her concussion have completely resolved. That means, using the first method, no athlete should be returned to play until his or her baseline symptom inventory score is equal to what it was prior to the start of the season. Using the second method, no athlete should return to play until his or her symptom score is equal to zero. Although reasonable exceptions to this rule may sometimes be made, they should be infrequent, and supervised by a clinician with expertise in the assessment and management of sport-related concussion.

Medications are often used to help treat the symptoms of an athlete who experiences a prolonged recovery from a sport-related concussion. Once the athlete is no longer experiencing these symptoms, medications should be discontinued. Some medications, however, cannot be stopped abruptly. Therefore, even though the athlete may no longer be experiencing symptoms from his or her concussion, the physician prescribing a medication will recommend the athlete continues to take it for some period of time. Often the medication will have to be tapered as opposed to abruptly stopped. When tapering off of a medication, an athlete decreases the daily dose slowly, over a period of days to weeks, until he or she is on such a small dose that it can be stopped safely. In order to be returned to sports safely, athletes must remain symptom-free even after the medication has been stopped.

Therefore, athletes who are still taking a medication to treat the signs and symptoms of concussion should not be returned to sports, even if they are symptom-free while on the medication. Exceptions to this rule, as always, should be made by clinicians with experience in the assessment and management of sport-related concussion.

Headaches are the most common symptom of sport-related concussion. There is even some evidence that athletes who sustain migraine like symptoms after concussion take longer to recover than other athletes. Recent medical investigations are considering whether athletes who have family members who suffer migraine headaches also take longer to recover from sport-related concussions than other athletes. These associations between migraine headaches and recovery from concussion have led some clinicians to believe that certain people, who may be predisposed to migraine headaches may also be predisposed to suffering sport-related concussions.

We all suffer headaches from time to time. Some people have very specific headaches that they suffer on a fairly regular basis. Many readers will know someone who suffers from migraine headaches. It is well known that trauma to the head can result in the onset of migraine headaches, even when the patient has not sustained a concussion, or when the patient has recovered from his or her concussion. Therefore, it can sometimes be unclear whether athletes are experiencing headaches because they are still recovering from their concussions, or whether they have headaches that were brought about by their trauma, and continue despite the fact that they have recovered from their concussions. Again, these decisions should be made by a clinician with expertise in the assessment and management of sport-related concussion.

As noted previously, many of the signs and symptoms of sport-related concussion can be seen in other illnesses or disease processes. The treatment of a sport-related concussion in and of itself can result in some symptoms. Sport-related concussions can result in irritability, depressed mood, low energy, and insomnia. However, the same symptoms can result from the treatment of sport-related concussions, namely, restrictions placed on physical and cognitive activities. Most athletes choose to participate in sports. Most of them enjoy playing sports. They enjoy exercising. Exercise improves their mood and overall sense of well-being. Since one of the treatments of sport-related concussions is physical rest, these athletes are removed from sports and exercise during their recovery. This often results in the onset of irritability, depression, and increased emotionality. Therefore, it can be difficult to determine, at times, whether the symptoms are due to incomplete recovery from a sport-related concussion or due to the treatment of sport-related concussion. In order to help distinguish between these two possibilities, doctors will occasionally allow an athlete to return to some safe, light, aerobic activity prior to full resolution of his or her symptoms. Oftentimes being allowed to exercise in such a manner will improve the patient's mood, as well as alleviate depression, help with difficulty sleeping and decrease their irritability. With the release of the new consensus statement allowing for a return to exercise somewhat earlier than previous statements of recommended, we will hopefully see a decrease in the effects on mood.

Regular exercise can also increase one's energy. Therefore, being removed from exercise can decrease one's energy. People who lead a sedentary lifestyle often complain of feeling fatigued, tired and having low energy. Regular exercise can improve these symptoms. Again, since athletes have been removed from exercise and physical activity during the recovery from sport-related concussions, decreased energy may result. Returning to some light aerobic activity in a safe setting can often improve their overall energy and help distinguish between incomplete recovery and the effects of physical rest.

While exercise can improve one's overall energy during the waking hours, physical exertion is also tiring. Therefore, many athletes will sleep well through the night, often requiring more hours of sleep then sedentary individuals. Once again the removal from physical exertion as part of treatment for a sport-related concussion can result in sleep disturbance or insomnia, which is a difficulty falling asleep or maintaining sleep. Insomnia, however, is one of the main symptoms of concussion. In particular, athletes who take longer than days to weeks to recover from their concussion will rank insomnia as one of their most significant symptoms. By allowing athletes to return to some light aerobic activity in a safe setting, their sleep can be improved.

In addition to symptoms, an athlete's balance is used to track his or her recovery and to determine when it is safe to return to sports. As noted in the previous section, many athletes will have a balance error system score recorded prior to the start of the season. After a concussion, athletes' balance is often worse. It improves as they recover, until they are just as steady on their feet as they were before the season started. An athlete should not be considered completely recovered until his or her balance has returned to pre-injury levels.

Again, some exceptions to this rule may be made. One can imagine athletes might sustain an ankle or knee injury at the same time as their concussions. They may recover from their concussions quite quickly. However, they may still have some residual injury to the ankle or knee. This may adversely affect their balance. Decisions to return athletes to play prior to full recovery of their preseason balance should be made by a clinician with expertise in the assessment and management of sport-related concussion.

Brain function is also used to assess recovery from a sport-related concussion. Most commonly the assessment of brain function is measured using computerized neurocognitive testing as discussed in previous chapters. Ideally, athletes will have measurements of their brain function prior to the start of the athletic season. In the event of a concussion, their brain function will be reassessed and compared to what it was prior to their injury. Any deficits from their preseason or baseline functioning should be considered reflective of injury. Athletes should not be returned to sport until their brain function has recovered back to its preinjury level.

The assessment of these neuropsychological scores can be somewhat complicated. Any time people take a test of any kind more than once, they are likely to get a different score than they did previously. People always do a little bit better or little bit worse than they did before. This is expected. Therefore, athletic trainers, doctors, neuropsychologists, and other people interpreting these computerized neuropsychological tests must take this normal background variation in scores into account. They must decide when a test score is so much better or so much worse than a previous test score that it represents true injury or true recovery as opposed to simply background variability. Methods of statistical analysis are used to assist in this determination.

Furthermore, performance on these computerized neuropsychological tests can be affected by many factors. If athletes are ill at the time of the test, they may perform worse than if they were healthy. Similarly, if they are tired at the time of the test, they will perform worse than when they are well rested. Athletes who are depressed may perform more poorly than they would if they were in good spirits. In addition, athletes will have different motivation. Those taking a preseason baseline test may not be motivated to do well, since there's nothing at stake. An athlete taking a post-injury test 10 days before a championship game, however, will be highly motivated to score well on the test. Likewise, some athletes may be participating in a sport that they do not particularly like. They may have little desire to return to that sport and therefore be less motivated when taking tests after injury than they would be if they enjoyed their sport. All of these factors must be taken into account by the clinician who is interpreting the scores.

As computerized neurocognitive tests become more common in the assessment and management of sport-related concussions, athletes become more familiar with the process and how these tests are used. Therefore, some athletes will intentionally do poorly on their preseason baseline. That way, if they sustain a sport-related concussion during the season, they might still be able to achieve their baseline scores, even while concussed. In this way, these athletes hope to be returned to sport prior to full recovery. They should be cautioned, however, that many of these computer programs have hidden mechanisms within the test that allow clinicians to determine whether the athlete put forth a good effort. Experienced clinicians will be able to decipher whether an athlete has purposefully performed poorly. Those athletes will be required to repeat the test prior to the being cleared for game play. In fact, investigators at Colorado College conducted a study with a instructed athletes to try and "sandbag" their computerized neurocognitive assessment while avoiding detection. Only 11 percent of athletes were able to do so.

Athletes should not be cleared to resume sports until they have reachieved their prior levels of brain function. Again some exceptions to this rule may be considered. Rarely, athletes may have the day of their lives when they take their baseline test. They may score much higher than they would on any other occasion. Therefore, some athletes who have had complete resolution of their symptoms, who have had complete return of their balance, and who remain symptom-free despite days or weeks of full participation in the noncontact activities of their respective sports may be cleared to return to play despite not having reachieved their preinjury neuropsychological test scores. Again decisions such as this should be made by clinicians with expertise in the assessment and management of sport-related concussion.

Recently, there has been some debate in the medical and neuropsychological literature regarding who should be interpreting these scores. Some feel that these computerized assessments should only be interpreted by a neuropsychologist. Others argue that these assessments are a relatively small part of neuropsychology, and other clinicians with different medical backgrounds can be taught to administer and interpret these scores reliably. As many concerned athletes, coaches, and parents may hear this debate, I will offer my opinion and some clarification here.

As a medical doctor I was trained to do many things. One of those things was to perform a physical examination of the patient. There are various components of the physical examination. The component of the physical examination that relates to the brain, the nerves, and the ability of brain function is known as the neurological examination. While learning the neurological examination medical students are taught how the normal body appears, how it reacts to certain stimuli, and how the ill or injured body reacts differently than the normal, healthy body. For example, many readers will recall a time when they were seen by a doctor and had a light shone in their eyes. The black circle in the center of people's eyes is known as the pupil. Light travels through the pupil to a nerve at the back of the eye that is connected to the brain. This is how we are able to see. The brain interprets the light that strikes this nerve at the back of the eye. When a bright light is shined into the eye of a normal, healthy patient, the pupil will become smaller or constrict. In certain disease processes or other states the pupil is abnormally small and will not constrict. In other disease processes the pupil is abnormally large and will not constrict. Sometimes the pupil of the left eye is a different size than the pupil of the right eye. This can be due to disease or injury. But it can also be a normal finding. Doctors have learned how to interpret these findings and determine whether they are normal, due to disease, or due to injury. This is one small part of the neurological examination. And the neurological examination is one small part of the overall physical examination. And the physical examination is a small part of the complete medical assessment that the doctor learns while going through medical school. While I do not think it is possible for someone to learn everything that is taught during medical education without going to medical school and completing a residency, I do believe that other clinicians can be taught to examine the pupil properly. Indeed, nurses, nurse practitioners, physician's assistants, and neuropsychologists themselves can be taught certain components of the neurological examination without learning the remainder of everything that is taught during medical school and medical residency.

Likewise, physicians, athletic trainers, nurses, and other medical personnel can be taught to administer and interpret computerized neurocognitive tests without having to complete the full training of a neuropsychologist. Certainly, there will be times when these computerized neurocognitive assessments will be difficult to interpret. At times like this, the opinion of a neuropsychologist should be sought. Indeed, where I work at the Sports Concussion Clinic in the Division of Sports Medicine at Children's Hospital Boston, we work very closely with many neuropsychologists on interpreting these scores. In addition, our neuropsychologists help us make the diagnosis of concussion, help determine when an athlete has recovered from a concussion, and provide academic planning for students who have significant brain dysfunction after sustaining a sport-related concussion. Neuropsychologists are an essential part of our sports concussion clinic.

The best approach for managing concussive brain injuries involves a team of personnel, including all of the various specialties and subspecialties mentioned in this book. However, not all athletic teams, hospitals, or other medical clinics will have access to neuropsychologists. Therefore, other medical professionals should be taught to administer and interpret computerized neurocognitive test scores for the limited purpose of assessing sport-related concussions and determining when an athlete has recovered. There are relatively few neuropsychologists in comparison to the number of athletic trainers, physicians, nurses, and other medical professionals combined.

Furthermore, some neuropsychologists who are well versed in the traditional types of neuropsychological testing will not be familiar with the computerized neuropsychological tests used for assessing sport-related concussions. Specific training on administering and interpreting computerized tests is necessary, even for neuropsychologists who trained only in the more traditional paradigms.

To ensure the highest quality of care is given to all athletes, other medical professionals need to be trained to administer and interpret computerized neuropsychological tests for the limited function of assessing sport-related concussion. Ideally, this would be in conjunction with a trained neuropsychologist to whom patients could then be referred for more in-depth analyses when necessary.

There are other modalities currently being investigated that might add additional information to the assessment of concussion and recovery from concussion. More than measuring balance, changes in gait, particularly changes in gait observed when the mind is distracted by doing other tasks, have been studied in the setting of sport-related concussion and may prove useful as a means of monitoring recovery. Furthermore, there have been a number of studies exploring the movement of the eyes and the ability of the eyes to follow objects in motion after concussion, generally termed ocular motor function. Several studies have shown changes in oculomotor function after concussion that resolve during recovery. The assessments of oculomotor function may also be useful in the future as a means of diagnosing and monitoring recovery from sport-related concussion.

While symptoms, balance, and neurocognitive function are the three main components in helping determine when an athlete has recovered from a sport-related concussion, there are many other factors that are considered before returning an athlete to sport. Even when an athlete has recovered fully from a sport-related concussion, medical professionals may recommend further avoidance of high-risk athletic activities for a period of time. Some of the other factors used to determine when an athlete can be put back to sport are discussed next.

NUMBER OF LIFETIME CONCUSSIONS

Although there is no absolute number of concussions after which an athlete should not return to contact sports, collision sports, or other high-risk athletic activities, most clinicians still take the total number of concussions an athlete has sustained during his or her lifetime into consideration when making decisions about returning to sports. In general a more conservative approach is warranted after an athlete has sustained several concussions compared to an athlete who has sustained only one or two. In other words, athletes who have sustained multiple concussions should be given more time to recover from their injuries before being returned to game play or other risky activities than athletes who have only sustained one concussion.

DURATION OF RECOVERY TIME FROM CONCUSSION

Many athletes will have full resolution of their post-concussion symptoms within a few days to weeks. In a study published in the *Journal of the American Medical Association* in 2003, 90 percent of college football players who sustained a sport-related concussion had resolution of their symptoms within 10 days. A study of high school athletes published in the *American Journal of Sports Medicine* in 2010 showed that nearly 85 percent of high school athletes who sustained a sport-related concussion had complete resolution of their symptoms and were deemed recovered by their athletic trainer within seven days after injury. Within one month after their injury, 98.5 percent of high school athletes who sustained a sport-related concussion were deemed recovered by their athletic trainer. However, some unfortunate minority of athletes will have symptoms that last much longer. Athletes who experience these prolonged recoveries are often held out of contact sports, collision sports, or other risky athletic activities for a longer period of time than those who recover more quickly. This is to allow the brain further time to heal before exposing it to another potential injury.

AMOUNT OF FORCE RESULTING IN CONCUSSIONS

We have all seen major collisions in American football or ice hockey that have resulted in an athlete suffering a sport-related concussion. For some athletes, however, especially if they have sustained prior sport-related concussions, a much lower level of force results in a concussive brain injury. If an athlete appears to be sustaining concussions with a progressively lower level of force, clinicians become concerned. Often, we will recommend a longer period of recovery even after symptoms resolve, balance is returned to normal, and brain function has recovered to baseline, before clearing such an athlete to return to their sport.

TYPE OF ACTIVITY OR SPORT TO WHICH THE ATHLETE WISHES TO RETURN

The type of activity or sport to which athletes wish to return is a key component in deciding when they may return. Tennis is a relatively low-risk sport as far as sport-related concussion is concerned. Therefore, an athlete might be returned to tennis almost as soon as he or she has recovered from a concussion. In fact, there may be situations where an athlete is allowed to participate in tennis while still recovering from a sport-related concussion. If that same athlete, however, wished to return to ice hockey, football or rugby, clinicians would mandate that their symptoms be entirely resolved, including with physical and cognitive exertion, and would often recommend a longer symptom-free waiting period. In some cases not only the sport the athlete wishes to play but also the position the athlete will be playing factors into decisions regarding return to play. For example, some clinicians will require a longer period of recovery for cheerleaders who are flyers, given the high-risk nature of their cheerleading activities, compared to other cheerleaders.

THE GOALS OF THE ATHLETE

Athletes' long-term goals play a major role in determining if and when they return to their sport. It is not uncommon for athletes who have sustained three or four concussions over the course of their lifetime to wish to return to their contact or collision sport. Those of us practicing medicine know that there is a risk of sustaining multiple concussions. The exact number that results in long-term problems is unknown. In fact, it is likely that there is no exact number. It is more likely that the number is different for each athlete, depending on the physical and biological characteristics of the athlete, the forces involved in each injury, and many other factors that we in medicine have not yet elucidated. Some athletes will sustain many concussions and not suffer any permanent or long-term problems. How long an athlete must wait before returning to sport after a concussion, or whether they should return to sport at all after sustaining multiple concussions, depends on their lifetime goals. If a junior in college who plays for the varsity team has sustained his third lifetime concussion, and his long-term goal in life is to become a veterinarian, he and his clinician may decide that the potential long-term risks of returning to sport and possibly sustaining a fourth lifetime concussion are not worth taking. However, if that same college junior plays for a high-level college program, aspires to play professional hockey in the National Hockey League, and given his current skill level, abilities, and reputation, this is a realistic possibility for him, he and his clinician may decide that he will return to sport and assume the potential risks of a fourth lifetime concussions.

Although some readers may see this as controversial, it is difficult to take away somebody's livelihood, his means of earning a living, over a potential risk that may or may not ever occur. Many athletes have sustained five, six, seven, or more concussions over the course of their lifetime without suffering any measurable permanent or long-term problems. Others may have problems after having sustained fewer concussions. Since those of us in medicine cannot accurately predict which number of concussions will lead to long-term problems, nor which athletes are at risk for these problems, each case must be decided individually with the aspirations, concerns, and understanding of the athlete in mind. Many times, conversations such as these will also involve all of the clinicians caring for the athlete, the athlete's loved ones, and the other important people in the athlete's life. Most often, the conversation takes place over a series of visits, lasting anywhere from several weeks, to months, or even years in some athletes who sustain multiple concussions over the course of their academic and professional careers.

THE SEVERITY OF COGNITIVE DEFICITS OBSERVED
AFTER CONCUSSION

Some athletes will not sustain measurable cognitive deficits in their brain function with their concussions. Other athletes will sustain mild deficits in their brain function with their sport-related concussions. Still other athletes will sustain marked and significant deficits in their brain function with their concussions. It is not uncommon for clinicians to recommend a longer time away from contact sports, collision sports, or other risky athletic activities for athletes who have sustained more dramatic deficits in their brain function after injury. For athletes who used to suffer relatively mild cognitive deficits with their first few concussions but are now suffering much more significant cognitive deficits after sustaining multiple concussions, the length of time prior to returning to contact or collision sports is often increased to allow for further recovery.

THE SEVERITY OF SYMPTOMS EXPERIENCED BY THE ATHLETE AFTER CONCUSSION

Some athletes will experience only mild symptoms as a result of their concussions. Others will experience more severe symptoms, even incapacitating symptoms. Most clinicians will recommend longer times away from sport for those athletes who have sustained more severe symptoms than for those who have only mild symptoms after their concussion. In addition, if athletes who sustained relatively mild symptoms after their first concussion now have more significant symptoms after sustaining multiple concussions, clinicians often recommend longer recovery times.

THE AGE OF THE ATHLETE

Usually, children recover more quickly from injuries than adults do. Concussion is one of the few injuries from which it seems adults recover more quickly than children. Medical studies conducted in older athletes have shown shorter recovery times after sport-related concussions than medical studies conducted in younger athletes. The reason for this is unclear. It could be that the younger, developing brain of pediatric athletes heals more slowly than the fully developed brain of more mature athletes. It could also be, however, that those athletes who require long times in order to recover from their sport-related concussions stop playing high-risk sports at a younger age. Thus, they are no longer at risk of sustaining a sport-related concussion. Lastly, it has to do with the difference in the methods used to conduct this study. Often the duration of recovery is measured at the time between injury and when the athlete is ultimately cleared to return to sports. Physicians may be more cautious when managing younger athletes, and therefore keep them out of sports for longer period of time despite the fact they have fully recovered. Furthermore, older athletes are more likely to play for a team with greater resources. Younger athletes often compete for teams that have no athletic trainer, no team physician, no emergency action plan, and no concussion protocol. These athletes have fewer baseline assessments available to help determine when they are recovered. Since it is often more difficult to determine when these athletes are fully recovered, longer recovery time is frequently recommended.

Until we know more about the recovery from a sport-related concussion and how recovery is affected by age, it is prudent to keep the pediatric athlete out of sports for a longer period of time than the older athlete.

OTHER FACTORS

There are many other factors that may contribute to the decision to return an athlete to sports. These decisions are complicated. Since the medical community has only recently begun to pay attention to sport-related concussions, there is much we do not know about them. There are no specific tests that can definitively diagnose sport-related concussions or determine precisely when recovery has occurred. While there is now evidence supporting the possibility that that some athletes will suffer long-term effects from sustaining multiple sport-related concussions, we do not yet have the ability to predict which athletes are vulnerable to these long-term effects, how many injuries are needed before one suffers these long-term effects, or what other factors might help predict which athletes are likely to develop these long-term problems. Until such information is available, doctors, athletes, parents, neuropsychologists, and all other people involved in the assessment and management of sport-related concussions must weigh the potential risks and benefits of each individual case prior to determining when it is safe for an athlete to return to contact sports, collision sports, or other risky athletic activities.

In summary, clinicians use athletes' symptoms, balance, and cognitive function to help determine when it is safe to return to sports after sustaining a sport-related concussion. Ideally, measurements of these factors are taken before the athlete sustains a concussion. When such data are available, most athletes should not be returned to sports until after they have reachieved their baseline levels. In the absence of such baseline measurements, longer recovery times are often recommended. Similarly, longer recovery times are recommended for younger athletes, athletes who have sustained multiple concussions, athletes with pronounced signs and symptoms after their concussions, athletes who sustain concussion after collisions involving minimal force, athletes with prolonged recoveries, as well as athletes with other concerning circumstances. In most cases, athletes should be off of any medication used to treat their post-concussion symptoms prior to being cleared for contact or collision. Since there is no medical test that can accurately determine when it is safe for an athlete to return to contact or collision sports after a sport-related concussion, clinicians use many factors to help estimate the appropriate time for resuming these activities.

SUGGESTED READINGS

Guskiewicz, K.M., et al. Cumulative effects associated with recurrent concussion in collegiate football players: The NCAA concussion study. *JAMA*, 2003, 290(19): 2549–2555.

Lau, B., et al. Neurocognitive and symptom predictors of recovery in high school athletes. *Clin J Sport Med*, 2009, 19(3): 216–221.

McCrory, P., et al. Consensus statement on concussion in sport: The Fifth International Conference on Concussion in Sport held in Berlin, October 2016. *Br J Sports Med*, 2017 [Epub ahead of print].

McCrory, P., et al. Consensus statement on concussion in sport: The 3rd International Conference on Concussion in Sport held in Zurich, November 2008. *J Athl Train*, 2009, 44(4): 434–448.

Meehan, W.P., III, P. d'Hemecourt, and R.D. Comstock. High school concussions in the 2008–2009 academic year: Mechanism, symptoms, and management. *Am J Sports Med*, 2010, 38(12): 2405–2409.

10

THE ETHICAL CONSIDERATIONS OF SPORTS PARTICIPATION: SHOULD CHILDREN BE ALLOWED TO PLAY A SPORT THAT CARRIES A HIGH-RISK OF CONCUSSION?

Tennis player Casey Dellacqua is a U.S. open and French open doubles finalist and grand slam champion in mixed doubles. In October 2015 at the China Open in Beijing, Dellacqua was playing against Yaroslava Shvedova when Shvedova put a shot straight down the line. Dellacqua reached out with her forehand to make the return, but lost her balance, dropped her racquet, and fell backwards, snapping her head toward the court and striking the back of her head against the ground. She cannot recall the remaining 10 minutes of that match. The next thing she remembers is being in the hospital in Beijing. Despite playing what is considered to be a safe sport, particularly with regards to concussions, Casey Dellacqua was concussed.

That's right: concussion is a risk even in sports like tennis, which are generally considered safe. Still, the risk is low in tennis and most athletes and their parents would agree that the benefits of participating in tennis outweigh any potential risks of suffering a concussion. Therefore, few athletes and few parents of athletes would hesitate to allow their child to play tennis because of a concern regarding concussion. As the risks of concussion in a given sport increase, however, some have a more difficult time determining whether the risks outweigh the benefits. This is especially true for those athletes playing collision sports such as football, boys' ice hockey, rugby, or boys' lacrosse, but also for contact sports such as girls' lacrosse, girls' ice hockey, soccer, and basketball among others, as they are at risk for suffering more than one concussion over the course of their athletic careers. In fact, concerns over the risks of sustaining a concussion or multiple concussions in sports that carry a relatively high risk have led to calls to ban certain sports or certain elements of sports, rather than allow athletes and their parents to decide for themselves whether to participate.

The benefits from sports participation are innumerable. Participation in sports by young athletes is associated with social, psychological, and medical benefits, many of which extend into adulthood, including improved self-esteem, better cardiovascular conditioning, higher academic and career achievement, and a decreased risk of obesity, heart disease, stroke, certain cancers, social problems, teen pregnancy, sleep apnea, mental health problems, suicide, and all-cause mortality. Sports participation improves their self-image. As noted earlier, children playing team sports learn to interact with their peers, to assist those who are less skilled, and to learn from those who are more highly skilled. They learn to cooperate and to lead.

Sports, however, also carry a risk of injury. When considering participation in a given sport, athletes and, for pediatric athletes their parents, must decide whether the benefits of participating outweigh the risks. Recently, given the risks of catastrophic injuries (defined as those resulting in permanent neurological injury or death), sport-related concussions, and the potential for cumulative effects from multiple sport-related concussions including chronic traumatic encephalopathy (CTE), some have called for a complete ban on American football or a ban on tackling in football for children and adolescents. A consideration of these injuries and whether such measures should be taken is in order.

It is worth remembering that well-conducted prospective cohort studies show that most athletes have full resolution of their concussion symptoms and are deemed recovered by their medical care providers within a week of injury, with more than 90 percent recovered within a month. Increased risks are incurred when an athlete is returned to sports, particularly contact sports, prior to full recovery. Numerous cases of massive cerebral edema resulting in catastrophic injury have been reported due to contact prior to full symptom resolution, particularly in young athletes, an occurrence known as second impact syndrome. These cases, however, are rare, representing a minute fraction of athletes participating in football. In fact, the risk of any catastrophic injury (not just second impact syndrome) occurring in football is rare, estimated to be 1.78/100,000 participants annually. In comparison to other sports, this risk is lower than that of boys' gymnastics (4.07/100,000 participants annually), girls' ice hockey (2.76/100,000 participants annually), and boys' ice hockey (2.35/100,000 participants annually) and slightly higher than that of girls' gymnastics (1.41/100,000 participants annually) and boys' lacrosse (1.28/100,000 participants annually).

Athletes are at particular risk for the potential cumulative effects of sport-related concussions. While concussions are a relatively rare event in most activities of daily living, and therefore unlikely to occur repeatedly in non-athletes, concussions are comparatively common in sports. Potential effects of repeated concussions have been documented, including among athletes. In order to reduce the risk of developing these cumulative effects, focused efforts and standardized methods for diagnosing, tracking, and monitoring recovery from sport-related concussions have been developed.

CTE is a diagnosis made by specific pathological findings in the brain at autopsy, particularly "an abnormal perivascular accumulation of hyperphosphprylated tau in neurons, astrocytes, and cell processes in an irregular pattern at the depths of the cortical sulci." As of yet, the proportion of neurobehavioral symptoms and findings attributable to these pathological findings remains unknown. Animal models, however, suggest that the formation of a particular conformation of tau, *cis*-tau, is associated with and, in fact, causative of some of the neurobehavioral sequelae. Nearly all cases of sport-related CTE have been described in athletes who have had long careers, lasting beyond college into professional sports. Even among former professional football players, the prevalence of CTE remains unknown. As few young athletes make it into professional football, the exposure to repeated head trauma sustained by most young football players is of a shorter duration than that of known cases of CTE. Furthermore, the forces involved in collisions between young football players are lower than those faced by professional athletes ultimately diagnosed with CTE.

Physical inactivity, is a much bigger problem facing today's youth than CTE, with the World Health Organization estimating that physical inactivity results in 3.2 million deaths annually. Banning football would remove an option for some athletes to reap the benefits of sports participation and regular exercise. Athletes choose to participate in sports in which they can be successful. They enjoy sports in which they can make a meaningful contribution. Those sports they do not enjoy, they quit. Removing football as a possible sport essentially takes an option away from some athletes. Those who would argue that young athletes could just choose another autumn sport need to think the process through. While undoubtedly some athletes who currently play football could be successful and enjoy other common autumn sports such as cross country and soccer, many could not. Those with a large powerful body habitus that gives them an advantage in football are at a distinct disadvantage in these other sports. In addition, simply removing the contact from football would change the game such that it favors endurance and speed, again placing these athletes at a disadvantage. It should be noted, this same body habitus places them at an even higher risk of many of the health conditions prevented by sports participation and regular exercise, including those that are much more common than CTE such as, high blood pressure, obesity, high cholesterol, sleep apnea, and diabetes, among others. These athletes are the ones with the greatest need for regular exercise. Taking away an option that allows them to get regular exercise increases their risks of these common disorders, for which they're already high risk, in a misguided effort to decrease the risk of something that they are unlikely to develop.

It would be preferable, therefore, to make football safer than to ban it altogether. It is unlikely, however, that the risk of injury will be completely eliminated. As with all sports, there will remain some quantifiable risk of injury. Ultimately, after considering the risks and benefits of a given sport, young athletes and their parents must decide whether they wish to participate. This process is individualized; the risk:benefit ratio is unique to each athlete and for each sport. Furthermore, the risk:benefit ratio may change over time as other interests develop, skills change or injuries accumulate. Thus, decisions to participate should be revisited. Some will feel that any risk of catastrophic injury is too high and therefore, limit their options to golf, tennis, swimming, and cross country running. Some will feel the risks of catastrophic injury associated with gymnastics are too high, but those associated with wrestling (0.92/100,000 participants annually) are acceptable. Still other parents will feel that the substantial benefits to their child offered by gymnastics outweigh the risks. Likewise, while some athletes will be able to derive the same benefits by running cross country as they do from football, they may decide that the risk:benefit ratio of football is too great. Others, however, will know that their child is unlikely to run cross country or play soccer or engage in some other form of regular exercise if the option of football is taken away. Thus, football should be available as an option for those who decide the benefits outweigh the risks. Athletes and their families should be allowed to decide for themselves whether to participate in American football or other sports with relatively high risk of concussion such as those noted earlier.

Recently, the principals of biomedical ethics have been used as a framework to discuss whether children should be allowed to participate in contact and collision sports. The field of biomedical ethics is vast. There are entire texts on this topic and I encourage all of those interested in this topic to consider reading them further. There are multiple courses on ethics at some of the greatest medical institutions in the world. Indeed many physicians spend their entire careers discussing topics of biomedical ethics. Clearly, it is far too much to cover in this book. By laying out some basic principles upon which the field of biomedical ethics is founded, however, we can facilitate the discussion for our purposes in this chapter.

Although there are many different approaches to biomedical ethics, one approach used in modern-day medical ethics has, at its foundation, four basic principles that are used for making decisions:

1. Respect for autonomy (respect for the decision-making capabilities of an autonomous person)
2. Nonmaleficence (the avoidance of causing harm)
3. Beneficence (ensuring health-related benefits to the person or persons involved)
4. Justice (ensuring that the benefits and risks involved are distributed fairly among persons and/or populations)

RESPECT FOR AUTONOMY

The principal of respect for autonomy has a longstanding and solid foundation in America and many other western civilizations. It rises from philosophical teachings of Immanuel Kant and John Stewart Mill, among others. It confirms the ability and fundamental right of a person to make choices and take actions based on their own personal values, personal beliefs, and free from influence from outside forces. In the area of sports participation, the codes of athletic governing bodies such as International Federation of Sports

Medicine and the American Medical Association emphasize the importance of respect for autonomy. International Federation of Sports Medicine code of ethics states, "the team physician must . . . not refuse an athlete the right to make their [sic] own medical decisions." Furthermore in the American Medical Association code of ethics, in the section discussing athletes' participation in sports states, "physicians should assist athletes to make informed decisions about their participation in amateur and professional contact sports which entail the risks of bodily injury." In America we allow people to make their own decisions regarding their health, even if the wishes of the patient go against the course of action the doctor perceives to be best. Patients are free to refuse treatments despite a doctor's recommendation. The patient is free to engage in habits that may increase the risk of medical conditions and avoid habits that would decrease their risk of medical conditions. In brief, the principle of respect for autonomy requires us to allow athletes, once informed about the risks of participation in their chosen sports, decide for themselves whether they wish to participate.

NONMALEFICENCE

Nonmaleficence is a long-standing principal in the tradition of western medicine and was expressed in the Hippocratic oath as, "I will use treatment to help the sick according to my ability and judgment, but I will never uses it to injure or wrong them." When a physician is treating a patient, providing medical care to an athlete, or deciding whether a particular athlete should be allowed to participate in sports, the principle of nonmaleficence calls for us to avoid the causation of potential harm caused by our treatment.

BENEFICENCE

Another principle of modern-day biomedical ethics is the principle of beneficence. The principle of beneficence mandates physicians caring for athletes provide benefits to the athlete; it emphasizes a moral obligation to act for the benefit of the athlete. As there are many benefits to participation in organized sports, including major health benefits, the principal of beneficence requires physicians to allow and even encourage participation in sports by their patients.

JUSTICE

The fourth and final principle of biomedical ethics we will be discussing is justice. The principle of justice underscores the need for fair and adequate distribution of goods and benefits among people. It mandates that when we are making decisions regarding participation in sports, that we are fair and just, that we write policies that result in just outcomes.

For the topic under consideration in this chapter, whether we should allow athletes, particularly children, to participate in sports that carry a high risk of concussion, it will be readily apparent that several of these biomedical principles come into direct conflict. The principal of beneficence demands that we encourage all athletes to participate in sports, as there are enormous benefits to one's health and physical function as a result of participation in organized sports. Sports, however, also carry a risk of injury. Therefore, according to the principle of nonmaleficence, which emphasizes the obligation of health care providers to avoid inflicting harm, health care providers should discourage our patients from participating in sports. Finally, the principal respect for autonomy mandates that the physician allow capable athletes to decide for themselves whether they wish to participate in organized sports and obtain the potential benefits while incurring the potential risks. If we have full respect for autonomy, the physician caring for athletes will simply inform them of the risks and benefits of the sports they are considering participating in and allow them to make the decision themselves without influencing their decision one way or the other. For pediatric athletes, this decision is made by both the athlete and his or her parents. The principle of autonomy, however, is in direct conflict with both the principle of beneficence and the principle of nonmaleficence, as it calls for the physician to simply educate a prospective athlete, the athlete's family, and allow the athlete to decide for him or herself.

It should be readily apparent to most readers, therefore, that it is not uncommon for ethical principles come into conflict. Ethical principles are neither absolute nor universal. They need to be balanced among the other ethical principles involved in making a given decision. They need to be interpreted in the context of the situation to which they are applied. There is no ethical principal that clearly takes precedence over the others in all situations. The balance of a given ethical principle must be weighed against the value of another. This is perhaps best described by Beauchamp and Childress as follows:

> As a person's interests in autonomy increase and the benefits for the person decrease, the justification of paternalism is rendered less likely; conversely, as the benefits for a person increase and the person's interests in autonomy decrease the plausibility of an act of paternalism being justified increases. Thus, preventing minor harms or providing minor benefits while deeply disrespecting autonomy has no plausible justification; but preventing major harms or providing major benefit while only trivially disrespecting autonomy has a highly plausible paternalistic justification. (Beauchamp and Childress, 1994: 259–325)

Let us take the discussion outside of the realm of sport-related concussion for a moment to discuss a more common example of sports injury. One of the most common injuries in sports is an ankle sprain. Ankle sprains most commonly occur when athletes invert or roll their ankles. This stretches and in some cases tears the fibers of the ligaments on the outside of the ankle. A ligament is like a strap that attaches one bone to another. In the ankle, it attaches the foot to the lower leg. When athletes roll their ankles, they stretch the fibers of these ligaments and sometimes tear those fibers. This makes the joint less stable. It allows for greater range of motion at the ankle then is allowed when the ankle is uninjured. Therefore, when athletes sprain their ankles a decision must be made as to whether they may continue to participate in their sports. When sprains are mild, one can imagine that the benefits of continuing to participate might still outweigh the risks. The ankle could be braced or taped by an athletic trainer and athletes might be allowed to continue to participate. Certainly, they will be at increased risk of doing further damage to the ankle joint by participating. Since most injuries to the ankle recover fully and readily, however, and the benefits of continued participation can be substantial, we can imagine that the benefits of continued participation might outweigh the risks. For example, if an athlete has spent years of training for one signature event for which they have recently qualified and are due to participate in a few days suffers a mild ankle sprain, the benefits of participating in this once in a lifetime opportunity might outweigh the risks of additional damage to the ankle. In this scenario, the athlete's interests in autonomy, allowing him or her to make the decision whether to continue in sports despite incurring greater risk of damage to the ankle, is likely greater than the potential harm that could be done to the ankle.

One can imagine, however, a different situation. Suppose the athlete described previously sustained a fracture of the ankle as opposed to simply spraining it. An ankle fracture might result in much greater instability of the ankle and a much greater potential for additional damage could be done to the ankle joint, resulting in long-term complications such as decreased range of motion, increased risk of severe inflammation and arthritis in the ankle, and much more debilitating long-term effects on physical function and mobility. In this case, even if the athlete wished to incur the risk and participate in sport, the interest in nonmaleficence might outweigh the interest in autonomy, because the risks are so great.

Whether or not we are fully aware of it, we weigh the risks and benefits of our choices on some level in many scenarios frequently. We often do so rapidly, as many people feel the answers are obvious. Cross-country running, for example, is a common sports offered in the autumn of academic sports years. The aerobic activity associated with regular cross-country running improves cardiovascular function, helps control weight, improves muscle tone, and associated with long-term health benefits including decreased risk of obesity, cardiovascular disease, depression, diabetes, high cholesterol, high blood pressure, suicide, drug use, team pregnancy, cigarette use, and many other factors. Running cross-country, however, is not without risks. Cross-country athletes are at increased risk of spraining their ankles, suffering stress fractures of the lower leg, suffering stress fractures of the foot, and multiple other injuries. Still, the benefits of running cross-country are vast and many of these injuries are self-limited and easily treated. Therefore, for most of the population, the benefits associated with regular long-distance running outweigh the risks. Most people choose to participate in cross-country running without a great deal of deliberation.

Perhaps a more difficult decision involves commuting by bicycle, particularly in the city. There are massive benefits associated with the regular moderate to vigorous aerobic activity associated with bicycling. They are very similar to those noted earlier for running cross-country. Since one of the leading causes of morbidity in America's obesity and decreased physical activity, the risks of which may be reduce substantially by regular bicycling, in addition to the benefits and cardiovascular health, psychological health, and many others, some may choose to commute by bicycle. Still, it is not uncommon in the city to hear stories of bicyclists who are injured or killed after being struck by a motor vehicle. Therefore, many potential bicyclists are reluctant to bicycle or at least commute by bicycle; they worry about the risks involved being struck by motor vehicle. One can imagine that this is a process that involves more deliberation and consideration than choosing to run cross-country. Many potential bicyclists will feel that the risks of being struck by motor vehicle, and possibly killed, outweigh the potential benefits. Furthermore, they may be amenable to participating in other forms of aerobic exercise such as swimming, running, or playing tennis that don't have the risk of being struck by a car. Therefore, they choose not to ride a bicycle. There is, however, a substantial proportion of city dwellers to choose to commute to work by bicycle. While it is true that they could choose to drive to work while engaging in an alternate form of exercise, many don't even if they intend to. Many do not find running as pleasurable as riding a bicycle. Many live so many miles away from work that, while bicycling is quite feasible, it would be prohibitive to run such a long distance. Many do not have access to a swimming pool or tennis court. Still others would simply choose not to participate in these sports even if they were not riding their bicycles. In addition, since one has to commute to work anyway, the increased time it takes by bicycle is relatively small in exchange for the vigorous aerobic activity associated with it. This is especially true when compared to driving or walking to a pool, swimming, then showering, drying, changing, and driving to work. Therefore, many people choose to take the risks involved in bicycling to work, as for them, the benefits outweigh the risks. This decision varies by individual. Many factors such as the availability of other forms of exercise, the enjoyment of other forms of exercise, the environment in which one will be cycling, whether there are protected bike lanes or bike paths for part of the commute, and other such things factor into the decision. Those considering whether they wish to bicycle to work go through the process, however subconsciously, of weighing the potential risks versus potential benefits and making their decision.

The same process of weighing the risks against the benefits should be applied when deciding whether children can participate in sports, including contact and collision sports, which carry a risk of injury that is often higher than that of noncontact sports. The sport of American football has received a lot of attention in this regard. It is difficult to read a newspaper, watch the news, or with into the radio today without hearing about the risks of concussion in football. Therefore, these risks are front and center in the minds of many athletes and parents. Many athletes and their parents decide that the risk of sustaining a concussion in football is too high compared to the benefits and therefore they choose not to participate. This will be particularly true if there are other sports offered during the same season with which they obtained equal enjoyment. Many other athletes and their parents recognize that, while football carries a relatively high incidence of sport-related concussion compared to other team sports, only 5 to 20 percent or so of players per season will suffer a concussion, meaning that 80 to 95 percent won't. For most of the players who do sustain a concussion, it will be a self-limited injury that will resolve within a few days to a few weeks. Many of these athletes would not enjoy the other sports that are offered during the fall season. Therefore, many consider the benefits of participating in football to outweigh the risks. Therefore, they decide to participate in football despite the risks of sport-related concussion. For personal stories on making this difficult decision please see the sections by Charlie Cook and his mother Dr. Maureen Cook in Chapter 17 of this book.

In summary, the decision as to whether children should be allowed to participate in certain sports, particularly those with a relatively high risk of concussion, should be based on the athlete's individual circumstances. Athletes and their parents should weigh the potential benefits of participating in football or any other sport against the potential risks. These risks should not be limited to sport-related concussion, but should include the risks of other injuries as well. They must decide for themselves as both the benefits and the risks are unique and vary from person to person and from family to family. The amount of risk one is willing to accept for a given benefit varies by person. Some people are risk averse and would prefer to forego many benefits in order to avoid incurring additional risk of injury. Other people are less risk averse and are willing to take on more substantial risks to derive the well-established benefits associated with organized sports participation. In some circumstances where the risks are great and the potential infringement on the respect for autonomy slight, options may be limited by governing bodies or medical personnel. In situations where the potential risk is trivial and the potential benefit is substantial, the respect for autonomy will outweigh the risks and the decision should be left entirely up to the athlete. In many situations, the answer is less clear and it is only through conversation and deliberation that an acceptable and ethical decision can be made. This is particularly true in athletes who have sustained many injuries or have complicated recoveries after their concussions.

SUGGESTED READINGS

Beauchamp, T. L., and J. F. Childress. *Principles of Biomedical Ethics*, 4th edition. Oxford: Oxford University Press, 1994.

Cantu, R. C. Second impact syndrome: A risk in any contact sport. *Phys Sportsmed*, 1995, 23(6): 27.

Chomitz, V. R., M. M. Slining, R. J. McGowan, S. E. Mitchell, G. F. Dawson, and K. A. Hacker. Is there a relationship between physical fitness and academic achievement? Positive results from public school children in the northeastern United States. *J School Health*, 2009, 79(1): 30–37.

Donnelly, J. E., and K. Lambourne. Classroom-based physical activity, cognition, and academic achievement. *Prev Med*, 2011, 52 (Suppl 1): S36–S42.

Fiuza-Luces, C., N. Garatachea, N. A. Berger, and A. Lucia. Exercise is the real polypill. *Physiology*, 2013, 28: 330–358.

Goldstein, L. B., et al. American Heart Association and nonprofit advocacy: Past, present, and future. A policy recommendation from the American Heart Association. *Circulation*, 22 2011, 123(7): 816–832.

Gronwall, D., and P. Wrightson. Cumulative effect of concussion. *Lancet*, 1975, 2(7943): 995–997.

Hainline, B., and R. G. Ellenbogen. A perfect storm. *J Athl Train*, 2017, 52(3): 157–159.

Harris, D. High school football ban proposal under attack in New Hampshire. 2012. http://abcnews.go.com/US/high-school-football-ban-proposal-attack-hampshire/story?id=17559475.

Haskell, W. L., et al. Physical activity and public health: Updated recommendation for adults from the American College of Sports Medicine and the American Heart Association. *Med Sci Sports Exerc*, 2007, 39(8): 1423–1434.

Kirkwood M. Guest commentary: In youth sports, brew worth outweigh risks. *Denver Post*, January 22, 2016.

LeFevre, M. L. Behavioral counseling to promote a healthful diet and physical activity for cardiovascular disease prevention in adults with cardiovascular risk factors: U.S. Preventive Services Task Force recommendation statement. *Ann Intern Med*, 2014, 161(12): 894–901.

Marar, M., N. M. McIlvain, S. K. Fields, and R. D. Comstock. Epidemiology of concussions among United States high school athletes in 20 sports. *Am J Sports Med*, 2012, 40(4): 747–755.

McAllister, T., and McCrea Michael. Long term cognitive and neuropsychiatric consequences of repetitive concussions in head impact exposure. *J Athl Train*, 2017, 52 (3): 309–317.

McDonald, J., and G. D. Myer. "Don't like kids play football": A killer idea. *Br J Sports Med* 2016 [Epub ahead of print].

McKee, A. C., et al. Chronic traumatic encephalopathy in athletes: Progressive tauopathy after repetitive head injury. *J Neuropathol Exp Neurol*, 2009, 68(7): 709–735.

Omalu, B. I., S. T. DeKosky, R. L. Minster, M. I. Kamboh, R. L. Hamilton, and C. H. Wecht. Chronic traumatic encephalopathy in a National Football League player. *Neurosurgery*, 2005, 57(1): 128–134; discussion 128–134.

Robbins, L. Let's ban tackle football under age 18. *Real Clear Sports*, December 6, 2012. http:// www.realclearsports.com/articles/.

Saunders, R. L., and R. E. Harbaugh. The second impact in catastrophic contact-sports head trauma. *JAMA*, 1984, 252(4): 538–539.

Vina, J., F. Sanchis-Gomar, V. Martinez-Bello, and M. C. Gomez-Cabrera. Exercise acts as a drug: The pharmacological benefits of exercise. *Br J Pharmacol*, 2012, 167(1): 1–12.

Zemper, E. D. Catastrophic injuries among young athletes. *Br J Sports Med*, 2010, 44(1): 13–20.

11

PREVENTION: WAYS TO PREVENT AN ATHLETE FROM SUSTAINING A CONCUSSION

Iron Mike Tyson was a veritable wrecking machine. I remember arguing with other kids in the neighborhood about whether we could live through an unobstructed punch from Mike Tyson. I still don't know the answer. And I don't ever want to find out.

On November 22, 1986, Mike Tyson defeated Trevor Berbick to become the youngest champion to ever win the heavyweight title. He was only 20 years old. Berbick, the heavyweight champion at the time, was well known as he was the last man to fight Muhammad Ali. On paper, the fight appeared fairly well matched. In fact, given his height and reach, Berbick appeared to have a slight advantage. Tyson weighed in at 221 pounds to Berbick's 218 pounds. Berbick was 3 inches taller at 6 feet 2 inches compared to Tyson's 5 feet 11 inches. This translated to Berbick having a significant advantage in reach. While Berbick was more mature, at 32 years old, Tyson was young at mere 20 years old. But, as the fight would prove, this was not an even match.

During the first round, Tyson struck Berbick in the head with several powerful blows. With 23 seconds remaining in the first round, Berbick stumbled after sustaining a hard right to the head. Tyson pounced. He landed several additional blows that caused Berbick to drop his hands, clearly stunned by the assault. But he managed to remain on his feet until the bell rang. He was overpowered by Tyson. Within the first few seconds of round two, Tyson landed a series of powerful right and left hooks that knocked Berbick to the canvas.

The round continued. To those of us watching, it appeared that Berbick was simply trying to remain on his feet and sustain the periodic bursts of power from the challenger. With 38 seconds left, Tyson landed a right to the body, then an uppercut to the head, followed by a left hook that knocked Trevor Berbick to the canvas. Berbick tried to stand a total of three times. But he could only stumble and fall back to the canvas. He was dazed, confused, disoriented, and off-balance.

Trevor Berbick was concussed.

With boxers being constantly at risk for sustaining concussions, it would be wonderful if there were some effective means of preventing a concussion. This chapter will discuss potential ways of preventing concussions sustained by athletes. The theories behind individual prevention strategies will be reviewed. On a larger scale, strategies used by larger athletic organizations will be discussed. The evidence against or in support of these strategies, when available, will be included.

Unfortunately, there is no scientific, medically proven way of preventing a concussion. However, the experience of experts in the assessment and management of athletes has led to several strategies that are likely to help reduce the risk of sustaining a sport-related concussion, the recovery time after a sport-related concussion, and the risk of suffering long-term sequelae after multiple sport-related concussions.

EDUCATION

There are many ways that education can reduce the risk of sustaining a sport-related concussion, as well as the risk of suffering long-term sequelae after sport-related concussions. It is thought that the risk of sustaining a sport-related concussion is higher after a recent concussion. This comes from studies conducted in college-aged American football players. One such study reported that athletes who sustained two concussions in the same season suffered their injuries within 10 days of each other. Therefore, educating athletes, coaches, and parents to avoid returning an athlete to play too soon after a concussion can reduce the risk of these second injuries.

Additionally, the risks of suffering long-term sequelae after sustaining multiple sport-related concussions may increase as the number of concussions sustained over an athletic career increases. By learning more about the potential long-term effects of sport-related concussions, we hope that athletes will be more likely to report their injuries, manage their injuries appropriately, and refrain from returning to play prematurely. In fact, a medical study published in the journal *Injury Prevention* in 2003 showed that athletes who undergo a concussion education program learn more about concussion and even change their actions by avoiding certain penalties after the concussion training.

Concussions are more likely to occur when an athlete does not see a hit coming. There are certain types of hits that are more likely to result in a concussion than others. Educating athletes to avoid these types of hits can reduce the number of concussions. One such way of educating athletes has been studied in youth ice hockey. As part of this effort, players are given talks, brochures, and watch an educational video about hitting from behind. Because a hockey player cannot see a hit that is coming from behind, this is a high-risk situation as far as sport-related concussion is concerned. In order to reduce hits from behind, some league has even placed an octagonal red stop sign on the back of player's jerseys to remind their opponents not to strike them from the back. Similarly, coaching athletes to be aware of what is taking place around them and what potential collisions are coming may help improve their collision anticipation and decrease their risk of concussion. As was discussed earlier, proper collision anticipation is associated with a decreased risk of concussion, while inadequate collision anticipation is associated with an increased risk of concussion.

Also included under the heading of education should be the teaching of proper technique. Purposeful heading in soccer is a commonly debated topic that can help illustrate the importance of teaching proper technique. Although there is inadequate medical and scientific data supporting the hypothesis that purposeful heading in soccer causes sport-related concussions, many people contend that it does. In response to this possibility, there are soccer organizations that have disallowed some younger athletes to engage in purposeful heading of the soccer ball. I believe that this approach does more harm than good, especially if it is not accompanied by the teaching of proper heading technique at a younger age. I would recommend that younger athletes use smaller and softer soccer balls in order to develop the skills necessary for proper heading of the soccer ball, even if it is not allowed during competition.

Heading a soccer ball requires timing. It requires leg, back, and neck muscle strength. It requires physical coordination. It requires coordination between the eyes watching the soccer ball approach and the muscles of the legs, back, abdomen, and neck used for purposefully heading the soccer ball. These skills are best developed at younger ages, when athletes can only generate a certain amount of momentum with their kicks and throw-ins. I do not think the first time an athlete attempts to purposefully head the ball should be when it is drilled in the air with the force that some older children are capable of generating. I would not want the first time an athlete attempts to purposefully head the ball to be after it is kicked 30 feet in the air and 40 yards downfield by a powerful and skilled 12-year-old goal keeper. Since they are not as capable as their older counterparts of generating high velocities when throwing or kicking a soccer ball, I believe it is better to learn the proper skills and techniques of heading a soccer ball at younger ages.

HEADS-UP PLAYING

Playing with the head up, constantly being aware of what is taking place around an athlete can reduce the number of unexpected body checks. Since most concussions occur when an athlete does not see the hit coming, keeping the head up and being aware can potentially reduce the risk of sustaining a concussion. When athletes see a hit coming, they are able to brace themselves for impact and absorb the force of impact in such a way that their risk of injury is reduced. As discussed previously, medical studies in youth ice hockey have shown that players who see a hit coming and are able to absorb the hit properly are less likely to suffer a sport-related concussion and those who are struck unexpectedly. A study published in the medical journal *Pediatrics* in 2010 showed that in young, adolescent ice hockey players an anticipated hit resulted in less severe head impacts than unanticipated collisions.

NECK MUSCLE STRENGTH

Strengthening the neck muscles of an athlete may reduce their risk of sustaining concussions. Although many readers will be pleased to have put physics behind them after graduating from high school or college, a brief refresher in a simple, fundamental concept of physics will go a long way in explaining why this is. As we have already learned, athletes sustain concussions after a force is applied to their head or after a force is transmitted to their head from a blow sustained somewhere else on the body. This force results in a spinning, or rotational acceleration, of the brain. It is this rotational acceleration that causes the concussion.

Some readers may recall from physics that mathematically force is equal to mass multiplied by acceleration. That is to say that when a given force is applied to an object, how quickly that object accelerates away from the force depends on its mass. This is often represented by the equation:

$$F = ma$$

where F represents the force of the collision, m represents the mass of the object, and a represents the acceleration of the object after impact. Although it can sound confusing when put into scientific or mathematical terms, this concept is a matter of common sense for most readers. Suppose, for example, that I were to punch a ball as hard as I can. In scientific terms, we would say that there is a force involved in the collision between my fist and the ball. After the punch, the ball would roll away from me. How rapidly it rolls away from me or accelerates away from me would depend on the mass of the ball. If I were to punch a tennis ball, it would accelerate very rapidly away from me. If, however, I were to punch a bowling ball, it would accelerate relatively slowly away from me. This is what is meant by the mathematical equation $F = ma$. After being punched, given the same amount of force, a ball with a lot of mass, such as a bowling ball, will accelerate slowly, whereas a ball with little mass, such as a tennis ball, will accelerate more rapidly.

Since it is the acceleration of the brain after a force is applied or transmitted to the head that results in a concussion, we can reduce the risk of sustaining a concussion by reducing acceleration. One way to reduce the acceleration after a given force has been applied is to increase the mass of the head. An athlete can effectively do this by flexing his or her neck muscles. The mass of the human head is approximately 5 kilograms (11 pounds). Say the average mass of a male adult athlete's body is approximately 85 kilograms (187 pounds). When an athlete does not see a blow to the head coming, the 5 kilograms of the head will accelerate very rapidly. If, however, athletes see the hit coming and instinctively flex their neck muscles, the head becomes rigidly attached to the body. Therefore, after the blow is delivered, the head and remainder of the body act as one unit. Instead of the 5 kilograms of the head accelerating away very rapidly, the 85 kilograms of the body accelerates away more slowly. By strengthening their neck muscles, athletes can attach their heads to their body, so to speak, more effectively. Combining this increased neck strength with collision anticipation will reduce the acceleration of the head after impact and thereby reduce the risk of sustaining a sport-related concussion.

Athletes can add the following simple strengthening exercises to their current resistance training in an effort to reduce their risk of sport-related concussions. As with all resistance training, particularly in pediatric athletes, emphasis should be placed on a proper and safe technique. Pediatric athletes who are unfamiliar with resistance training should be coached and supervised by an adult with expertise in resistance training of the pediatric athlete. The following descriptions are solely for the purpose of describing the exercises available to the reader. Anyone planning to engage in these exercises should consult a proper manual or seek professional assistance.

1. **Shrugs**. Shrugs are a common resistance exercise and will be familiar to many readers. They can be performed using either a barbell or dumbbells. Perhaps the easiest way to do shrugs is for the athlete to have a dumbbell of appropriate weight in each hand. The arms are extended at the side. The athlete raises his or her shoulders lifting the weight of the dumbbell and then slowly relaxes to the starting position.
2. **Dumbbell press**. For the dumbbell press, the athlete has his or her arms raised so that the elbow is even with the shoulder on either side. The elbow is flexed to approximately 90 degrees. From this starting position, the athlete raises the dumbbell toward the ceiling while straightening the elbow. Then, the dumbbell is returned to the starting position.
3. **Lateral, forward, backward, and rotational resistance exercises of the neck**. Athletes playing for teams with significant resources will often have a machine that is designed to help them strengthen the muscles of their neck. However, there are some very simple resistance exercises that athletes without such resources may perform. Perhaps the easiest and one of the most effective ways of strengthening the neck muscles are these resistance exercises. In order to perform lateral resistance exercises, an athlete places his or her right hand along the right side of the head. The muscles of the neck are flexed such that the right ear attempts to move down toward the right shoulder. However, since the athlete is resisting this action, there is no actual movement of the head. The athlete should hold this position in active resistance for approximately 5 to 10 seconds. The exercise can then be performed on the left side of the head, front of the head, and back of the head. These exercises are known as the lateral, forward, and backward resistance exercises.

The rotational resistance exercises are similar. In order to perform this exercise the athlete would place his or her hand against the side of the forehead. The athlete then attempts to rotate the head toward the right or the left as when nodding "no." This motion is resisted by the hand. So there is no actual movement of the head. Again, the athlete would hold for a five or 10 second count and then repeat in the opposite direction.

GENERAL CONDITIONING AND STRENGTH

Although I am aware of little evidence to support this statement, I believe that the stronger and faster an athlete is, the less likely the risk of injury. This is not only true for the concussion but for all types of sports injuries. It will not be too difficult for the reader to imagine that a smaller, weaker, deconditioned athlete is at higher risk for injury than a bigger, stronger, faster athlete. The ability to dodge a blow from one's opponent or properly absorb a blow from one's opponent will decrease the risk of sport-related concussion. These abilities come with strength, conditioning, agility, and practice and experience.

CONFIDENCE

In addition to being recovered from a sport-related concussion, athletes should be confident that it is time for them to return to sport. They should be without fear. This is especially true for collision sports. There are few easier ways for an athlete to become injured than to be timid or hesitant. Opponents can tell when an athlete is timid. Any slightest hesitation will serve as an opportunity to deliver a controlling blow. An athlete who is worried about sustaining another injury and is afraid while on the field or ice does not have his or her head in the game. When your head is not in the game, you're more likely to be injured. Therefore, after athletes have recovered from sport-related concussions, emphasis should focus on retraining them and getting them ready for the demands of their sport before returning them to play. When athletes return to play after sport-related concussions, they should be fast, agile, and strong. They should have no fear. They should have no concerns. They should be confident. If they are not, consideration should be given to a further symptom-free waiting period, without contact, while they work through some of these issues.

PADDING AND EQUIPMENT

Many concussions, particularly in pediatric sports, occur after a collision between the player and an object, such as the goalpost in football. Proper padding around such structural objects may reduce the amount of force delivered at the time of these impacts and thereby reduce the risk of sport-related concussions. Similarly, age-appropriate equipment may reduce the risk of sport-related concussions. A common example of this can be seen in soccer. Oftentimes, younger athletes are seen playing soccer using an adult, regulation-sized soccer ball. Given the small mass of the pediatric athlete's head and body compared to that of an adult, the mass of the soccer ball used in play should be reduced.

ENFORCING THE RULES OF THE GAME AND DISCOURAGING DANGEROUS PLAY

While perhaps not always intentional, many concussions occur as a result of dangerous or illegal play. Body checks from behind in ice hockey, spear tackling to the helmet in football, dangerous kicks in soccer, elbows to the head and basketball, after play roughhousing in rugby can all result in a concussion. In fact, some medical studies conducted in junior league professional ice hockey have shown that many concussions result from illegal play. Unfortunately, this illegal play is not always noted by the referees. In addition to the education noted earlier, consistent and diligent enforcement of the rules and regulations of the game may be one of the most effective ways of reducing the risk of sport-related concussions. Some studies have shown but that by including penalty minutes in part of team rankings and decisions about postseason play, the number penalties and risk of injuries decreases. Perhaps when it comes to determining team rank we should not only consider teams' win-loss record, but also factor the number of penalty minutes they have been given throughout the season.

In summary, there are few medically proven ways of reducing an athlete's risk of sport-related concussion. However, educating athletes about the risks of dangerous play and the risks of returning to play before full recovery from a concussion may reduce the number of injuries and long-term consequences. Playing with the head up and being aware of one's surrounding may help prevent sport-related concussions. Athletes should not be returned to play until they are confident and ready to return to play with their "head in the game." General strengthening, conditioning and the strengthening of an athlete's neck muscles may help decrease his or her chance of sustaining a sport-related concussion. Attention to proper placement, padding, and securing of goalposts, netting, and other structures on the surface of play may reduce the risk of concussive brain injury. Proper rule enforcement can change athlete behavior, and result in a safer environment.

SUGGESTED READINGS

Cook, D.J., et al. Evaluation of the ThinkFirst Canada, Smart Hockey, brain and spinal cord injury prevention video. *Inj Prev*, 2003, 9(4): 361–366.
Guskiewicz, K.M., et al. Cumulative effects associated with recurrent concussion in collegiate football players: The NCAA Concussion Study. *Jama*, 2003, 290(19): 2549–2555.

Mihalik, J.P., et al. Collision type and player anticipation affect head impact severity among youth ice hockey players. *Pediatrics*, 2010, 125(6): e1394–1401.

Patlak, M. and J.E. Joy. Is soccer bad for children's heads: Summary of the IOM workshop on neuropsychological consequences of head impact in youth soccer. The IOM Workshop on Neuropsychological Consequences of Head Impact in Youth Soccer, 2002, National Academy of Sciences, Washington D.C.

Roberts, W.O., J.D. Brust, B. Leonard, and B. J. Hebert Fair-play rules and injury reduction in ice hockey. *Arch Pediatr Adolesc Med*, 1996, 150: 140–145.

Shewchenko, N., et al. Heading in football. Part 2: Biomechanics of ball heading and head response. *Br J Sports Med*, 2005, 39 (Suppl 1): i26–i32.

Shewchenko, N., et al. Heading in football. Part 3: Effect of ball properties on head response. Br *J Sports Med*, 2005, 39 (Suppl 1): i33–i39.

Viano, D.C., I.R. Casson, and E.J. Pellman. Concussion in professional football: Biomechanics of the struck player—part 14. *Neurosurgery*, 2007, 61(2): 313–327; discussion 327–328.

12

THE CUMULATIVE EFFECTS
OF CONCUSSION: HOW MANY
IS TOO MANY?

The story of former National Football League defensive back Andre Waters has become infamous throughout the field of sports medicine. Waters played during the 1980s and 1990s for both the Philadelphia Eagles and Arizona Cardinals. Over the course of his 12-year professional career, Waters was known as a hard hitter. His reputation earned him the nickname "Dirty Waters." He sustained many concussions during his career. In fact, during an episode of HBO's *Real Sports with Bryant Gumbel*, former Harvard University football player and professional wrestler turned concussion-in-sports activist Christopher Nowinski described Waters's concussion history as, "probably the worst concussion history that I've come across in any player."

After retirement, Waters suffered from numerous problems. He had a steady decline in his social and cognitive functioning. His memory was severely impaired. He suffered from depression. His emotions became uncontrollable. Ultimately, on November 20, 2006, several days before Thanksgiving, Andre Waters took his own life by a self-inflicted gunshot to the head.

His brain was sent to Pennsylvania pathologist, Dr. Bennet Omalu. Although Waters was only 44 years old at the time of his suicide, his brain had many similarities with that of older men. In fact, some of the medical findings discovered in Waters's brain were similar to that in patients suffering from Alzheimer's disease. After examining several similar cases, Dr. Omalu and others concluded that multiple concussions or head traumas sustained during their football careers led to their later life problems and the findings in the brains at autopsy. This story has recently been made into the movie the *Concussion* starring Will Smith.

In this chapter, we will review the studies suggesting cumulative effects of multiple concussions. The interpretation of the data will be discussed. The limitations of the data, given the recent changes in management of this injury, will also be discussed. Some guidance in determining when an athlete ought to consider retiring from collision or contact sports will be offered. A discussion of chronic traumatic encephalopathy (CTE), a more recent diagnosis made in several former NFL players, will be reviewed.

In the Sports Concussion Clinic in the Division of Sports Medicine of Children's Hospital Boston, athletes and their families often want to know whether it is safe to return to sports after a concussion. "How many is too many?" they often ask. This is a difficult question to answer. There are only a few medical studies that have investigated this question. The results are difficult to interpret because the way in which we diagnose concussion and manage athletes who sustain concussions has changed substantially over the last 10 to 20 years. This chapter will discuss some of the ways in which this question can be addressed.

Some clinicians say that athletes who have sustained three or more concussions over the course of their lifetime should be removed from contact and collision sports. Although I disagree with this practice, it is not entirely unreasonable. It is based on some medical evidence. Several studies have asked former athletes whether they have ever sustained a sport-related concussion. Those who answered "yes" were asked how many they had sustained over the course of their lifetime. Then, measurements were taken of their brain function. These studies showed that those athletes who reported they sustained three or more concussions during their lifetime performed worse on the assessment of brain function than those athletes who reported never sustaining a concussion. They suffered more symptoms and had more subjective memory problems than those who reported fewer concussions. Thus, many medical professionals feel that after three concussions, athletes should retire from contact and collision sports, since these sports carry the highest risk of concussion.

Indeed, this will seem like a very reasonable recommendation to most readers. But before reaching such a conclusion, let us consider some aspects of these studies. Most of the former athletes questioned played sports in the 1960s through the 1980s. Those readers who were also playing sports at that time will recall that the diagnosis and management of concussions was much different. In order to be diagnosed with a concussion back then, an athlete had to be knocked unconscious for so long that the game had to stop and the athletic trainer had to come onto the field and tend to the athlete.

Nowadays we know that 90 percent of concussions in sports do not involve a loss of consciousness. Nowadays, we diagnose athletes who sustain a rapid acceleration of the head followed by confusion, disorientation, nausea, headaches, imbalance, dizziness, and slowed speech with a concussion. Back then, such athletes were not routinely diagnosed with a concussion. They were simply told that they "got their bell rung," were "shaken up on the play," "got a ding," or they "got a dinger." Therefore, it is likely that many of the athletes in those studies who reported having three concussions may have sustained many more concussions by today's standards.

Similarly, the management of concussion has changed considerably. During the 1960s through the 1980s, athletes who sustained a sport-related concussion were often returned to play while still suffering from the symptoms of their concussion, many on the same day of their injury. In fact, most were returned to the game only a few minutes later. Missing a game or practice after a concussion was uncommon. Therefore, the poorer brain function, or "cognitive dysfunction," noted in these studies may not reflect the total number of injuries they sustained but rather the fact that they sustained multiple injuries before they were fully recovered from previous injuries. Nowadays, we no longer return athletes to play while they are still experiencing symptoms from a concussion.

In addition, these studies are susceptible to what is known as recall bias. Recall bias is a commonly described and fundamental factor that must be considered when conducting and interpreting medical research. As in the studies noted previously, it is common to ask people in a population about their exposure to some risk factor that occurred years prior to this study. In the examples noted, former football players were asked how many concussions they sustained during their years of active play. Recall bias refers to the phenomenon where people with a disease or medical condition recall their exposure to a risk factor differently than people without a given medical condition. Given the abundance of media publicity surrounding sport-related concussions and their potential for long-term effects, it is quite possible, even probable, that former athletes who now have cognitive difficulties are likely to attribute their problems to injuries they sustained during sports. They are likely to recall sustaining more concussions than a former athlete who is having no cognitive difficulties. Those now having cognitive difficulties may overestimate their exposure. This is true even when the exposure to the risk factor is similar between those with a given medical condition and those without.

The field of medicine has not yet figured out how many concussions is too many. In fact, it is likely no number exists. The number of concussions that leads to permanent deficits in memory, concentration, and other cognitive processes is likely to be different for each athlete. The number that increases the risk of dementia and other problems later in life is also likely different for each person. It might depend on the timing of the concussions with respect to one another. It might depend on the genetic makeup of the athlete. It might depend on the amount of force involved with each injury. And there may be many other factors involved that no one has yet considered. As we shall see later, the overall number of concussions an athlete has sustained still plays a role in making decisions about whether the athlete should return to contact or collision sports. But it is not the only factor or even the main factor in making such a decision. And there is no magic number after which physicians caring for athletes mandate retirement. For some athletes, the recommendation to retire from collision or contact sports might be made after only one or two concussions. Other athletes might be cleared to return to play after six or more concussions.

So if there is no magic number, how can you decide when an athlete has sustained too many concussions and should consider retiring from contact or and collision sports?

Several other factors besides the overall number help make this decision. Many of these are the same factors discussed earlier when deciding when it is safe to return an athlete to play after a sport-related concussion. For the sake of completeness, they will be reviewed again here.

Force: For some athletes, as the number of concussions they sustain increases, the force required to produce a concussion seems to decrease. For example, many athletes will report that their first concussion was sustained by a high force mechanism, such as a motor vehicle accident or a major blow delivered directly to the head by a larger opponent. Their second concussion was sustained by a more moderate force, such as a blow during a body check in ice hockey that witnesses recall as being a "big hit." But after the first several concussions, many athletes report developing symptoms after an accidental blow to the head by the arm of an opponent or friend. This is a concerning sign, and will prompt clinicians to discuss retirement form contact or collision sports with the athlete.

Slower recovery: Most athletes will recover from their concussions quickly, in a matter of days to weeks. As we have discussed earlier, in college aged athletes 90 percent of would-be completely symptom-free within 10 days of their injury. In high school aged athletes, nearly 85 percent will be symptom-free within one week of their injury. For some athletes, however, the recovery is markedly longer, lasting weeks to months. For others, they recover from their first one or two concussions quickly, just as most athletes do. But as they sustain more concussions, the recovery time increases, lasting weeks to months, or in some rare cases, longer than a year. This is another concerning sign that will prompt many physicians to discuss retiring from contact or collision sports with the athlete.

Pronounced cognitive losses: As discussed previously, cognitive function refers to one's ability to think, remember, concentrate, and reason. After a concussion, most athletes lose some of their cognitive function. As they recover, they regain their cognitive abilities. Full reattainment of cognitive function is one of the requirements for returning to play. For some athletes, the cognitive losses they experience at the time of injury increase as the number of concussions increases. That means, their memory, reaction time, and the speed with which they process information become markedly worse after their fourth concussion than it was after their first. This is another concerning sign that often prompts physicians to recommend retirement.

Similarly, some athletes will regain their cognitive function very quickly after first one or two concussions. However, as the overall number of concussions they sustain throughout their lifetime increases, the amount of time required for them to regain their cognitive function after injury also increases. When this occurs, many physicians will raise the issue of retiring from contact or collision sports with the athlete.

The decision to retire an athlete from contact or collision sports is a complicated one. For most athletes, retiring from these sports has a major impact on their lives. For professional athletes, their means for earning a living is taken away. For amateur athletes and college athletes trying to make the professional leagues, they have to give up their dream of playing in the pros. They have to choose another career. For college athletes without professional aspirations, high school athletes, and younger athletes, much of their social activity, self-identity, and enjoyment comes from their participation in contact or collision sports. Their physical health is improved by participation in sports. Many clinicians, parents, teachers, and other adults underestimate the importance of sports participation in young people's lives. Often, when athletes stop playing contact and collision sports, they lose their friends. This is most often unintentional. But most of the contact these athletes have with their friends is before practice, while dressing for sports, stretching, warming up, after practice while changing and showering, and on the bus ride to games. If concussed athletes are not around during these times, they miss out on conversations, jokes, the latest gossip, and the discussions that make people friends. This can be quite devastating. For more personal insight into the effects of removing an athlete from sport, please see the essays included in this book by Charlie Cook and his mother.

In the Sports Concussion Clinic of the Division of Sports Medicine at Children's Hospital Boston, the decision is most often made jointly, after a long discussion between the athlete, the athlete's family, other people important to the athlete, and the doctor. Often, the conversation involves a neuropsychologist and other members of the care team. This conversation takes place over a series of visits and lasts weeks to months. It is usually initiated after one of these findings has been noted: (1) less force seems to be required to produce a concussion; (2) the athlete appears to take longer to recover from successive concussions; (3) the athlete has more prolonged cognitive deficits after concussions than previously; or (4) the athlete has sustained many concussions. If none of these factors applies the athlete or, for younger athletes, the athlete's parents will often initiate the conversation by asking, "How many concussions is too many?"

I tell the athlete and others involved:

1. There is some risk of long-term problems after multiple concussions.
2. No one knows how many is too many.
3. The number is likely different for each athlete.
4. We will monitor the athlete for the factors noted earlier, and if they occur, we need to discuss possible retirement.
5. Athletes must understand that, even without the factors discussed earlier, there remains some risk.
6. They must decide for themselves whether they are willing to take that risk.

For athletes who earn their living by playing professional sports, most will accept a certain amount of risk and will continue to play after several concussions.

For those young athletes who do not seek to play professional sports, or who do not have a realistic chance of playing professional sports, most will assume less risk and will retire from high-risk sports after fewer concussions.

Ultimately athletes make the decision to retire themselves. On rare occasions, when the risk of returning seems too great, clinicians will refuse to allow an athlete to return against his or her wishes. But this is rare. In fact, of the thousands of athletes we have cared for in the Sports Concussion Clinic, I cannot think of a single case where an athlete was forced to retire from collision or contact sports against his or her wishes as a result of concussions. Even when I cannot personally clear the athletes to return to sports, I will offer them a second opinion with one of the other experts in the area.

What are all the news stories I see regarding professional athletes and concussion about?

Recently, there has been a flurry of media activity surrounding retired professional football players who have suffered dementia and other problems years after retirement. It is suspected that many of these problems resulted from their years in football, either as a result of sustaining multiple concussions, or as a result of sustaining multiple blows to the head that did not result in concussions, so-called subconcussive blows.

For a long time, people have suspected that multiple blows to the head might be bad for brain function. Indeed, many readers will recall statements about certain athletes in the past, meant as a joke, such as "that guy took one too many knocks to the head." While often said in jest, these types of statements, as with most jokes, may have had some element of truth to them.

Some physicians have also suspected that multiple blows to the head could cause problems. Dr. Martland's aforementioned article in the *Journal of the American Medical Association* in 1928 discusses a condition in boxers that he termed "punch drunk." Later, this same entity came to be known by the more medical-sounding term, "dementia pugilistica." Boxers suffering from dementia pugilistica had difficulties with memory, thinking, and concentration. They walked abnormally with a distinct dragging of the foot or leg. They often spoke slowly, and had notable changes in their faces.

The retired football players currently being discussed in the media have been diagnosed postmortem with an entity known as CTE. In 2005, in the medical journal *Neurosurgery*, a doctor by the name of Bennet Omalu, described the case of a retired National Football League Player who exhibited much of the same findings as boxers suffering from dementia pugilistica. After death, this former football player underwent an autopsy. His brain was notably different from that of a normal, healthy person. As he had no known trauma or blows to the brain except for those that he experienced while playing football, these changes in the brain were attributed to injuries he sustained while playing football. Since that time many other cases have been described by Dr. Omalu and others. Here in Boston, a group known as the Center for the Study of Traumatic Encephalopathy studies the brains of deceased, former athletes suspected of suffering from CTE. They have published the results of many cases of this condition. They have discovered that it is not exclusive to football players or former professional athletes.

It is not clear exactly what causes CTE. Certainly, it seems to be related to repeated blows to the head. Many of the athletes first noted to have CTE sustained multiple concussions over their careers. This led doctors to believe that CTE resulted from multiple concussions. However, CTE has since been discovered in athletes who were not known to have suffered many concussions. It is possible that these athletes sustained multiple concussions and simply did not tell anyone about them and therefore there is no record of these concussions. But it also raises the possibility that CTE does not result from the multiple concussions, but rather, from the hundreds or thousands of blows to the head that boxers and football players routinely sustain that do not cause a concussion. During nearly every play, the head of a lineman playing American football collides with the head of his opponent. Most of these blows do not cause a concussion. But perhaps they result in some small amount of injury to the brain that, when repeated thousands of times over the course of a career, ultimately leads to CTE. Similarly, boxers sustain many punches to the head over their careers. Most of these punches do not result in a concussion. But perhaps each punch, even when it does not cause a concussion, results in some small amount of injury to the brain that, when repeated thousands of times over the course of a boxer's career, leads to CTE.

Of course, there may be other factors involved. There are many football players and boxers who do not develop the proposed clinical signs and symptoms of CTE, and who have not had the pathological findings that define CTE, even after years of play. We do not yet know what the difference is between those who develop CTE and those who do not. Some studies have suggested that it may be due to genetic factors; some athletes may be predisposed to developing CTE after injury when compared to others. It may be due to environmental factors. Athletes taking certain medications, nutritional supplements, ergogenic aids or vitamins may be at higher risk of CTE than others. It may have to do with the timing of the injuries; perhaps injuries sustained close together are more likely to produce these findings then injuries sustained further apart. Perhaps sustaining repeated blows to the head at a certain age results in CTE whereas at other ages it does not. Or, it might not be related to any of these factors. In fact, it might not be due to trauma at all. Recently there have been studies not of professional athletes, soldiers, or others at risk for repeated trauma to the brain, but rather, average citizens who have passed away. When the brains of these average citizens are studied for the protein used to define CTE, approximately 35 percent of people have it. The proportion of people with this protein, known as hyperphosphorylated tau, is higher if they have a history of head trauma. But even in the absence of head trauma, the proportion of people carrying this protein is higher if they have abused substances, including alcohol. Even in the absence of head trauma and substance abuse, approximately

20 percent of people in this study stained positive for this protein. In addition, other case reports of people with no history of trauma or substance abuse but deposits of this abnormal protein in the same areas of the brain are emerging. Therefore, the cause of the protein is unclear. It may be that many factors increase the risk of developing it. Still, given the fact head trauma was associated with hyperphosphorylated tau in this study, and that animal studies show that trauma, in the absence of alcohol or other substances, will induce the abnormal form of the protein tau, cis-tau, it is likely the trauma is at least one risk factor associated with CTE.

It remains unclear, however, whether the protein causes the signs or symptoms that are currently being attributed to it. Some of those diagnosed with CTE at autopsy had successful post career lives and did not exhibit many symptoms or signs of brain disease. Furthermore, there are many people who suffer from headaches, depression, and memory problems later in life that were not exposed to repeated head trauma earlier in life. Therefore, larger studies with more participants will need to be conducted before the entity known as CTE is fully understood. Researchers are actively trying to determine which factors place athletes at risk for CTE so that we can better prevent and manage this disease.

Regardless of what we know or do not know about CTE, I think most people agree that there is no benefit to repeated trauma to the brain in sports. Repeated trauma to the brain neither benefits the athletes involved nor the game itself. Therefore, regardless of whether this protein results directly from trauma, regardless of whether this protein is directly responsible for signs and symptoms later in life, efforts to decrease the frequency of repeated trauma to the brain in sports should be undertaken.

In summary, for some athletes, multiple concussions may lead to a loss of some cognitive function that is not recovered. Some athletes who sustain multiple concussions over the course of their athletic careers will have problems later in life, including decreased cognitive abilities, dementia, mood disorders, headaches, and insomnia. The number of concussions that ultimately leads to long-term problems is unknown, and likely differs between athletes. It is likely that some athletes will sustain multiple concussions, and not have long-term problems. Still others may sustain long-term problems, after fewer sport-related concussions. And of course, there are people who, later in life, suffer from headaches, dementia, and other long-term problems who never sustained a concussion or played a sport that carries a high risk of concussion. Currently, there is no way for clinicians to tell which athletes are at risk for suffering problems later in life. There are likely multiple factors involved, including the number of injuries, the amount of force with each injury, and some underlying predisposition for long-term problems after a concussion in certain athletes. Until more is known, athletes should consider their own potential for personal risk, the importance of high-risk sports in their lives, and their long-term career goals when making decisions to return to contact sports, collision sports, or other high-risk activities.

SUGGESTED READINGS

Cantu, R.C. Chronic traumatic encephalopathy in the National Football League. *Neurosurgery*, 2007, 61(2): 223–225.

Gao, A.F., et al. Chronic traumatic encephalopathy-like neuropathological findings without a history of trauma. *Int J Pathol Clin Res,* 2017, 3: 50.

Guskiewicz, K.M., et al. Association between recurrent concussion and late-life cognitive impairment in retired professional football players. *Neurosurgery,* 2005, 57(4),. 719–726; discussion 719–726.

Guskiewicz, K.M., et al. Cumulative effects associated with recurrent concussion in collegiate football players: The NCAA Concussion Study. *JAMA,* 2003. 290(19): p. 2549–55.

Guskiewicz, K.M., et al. Recurrent concussion and risk of depression in retired professional football players. Med Sci Sports Exerc, 2007. 39(6): p. 903–9.

Kuhn, et al. Sports concussion research, chronic traumatic encephalopathy and the media: Repairing the disconnect. *Br J Sports Med,* 2016 [Epub ahead of print].

McKee, A.C., et al. Chronic traumatic encephalopathy in athletes: Progressive tauopathy after repetitive head injury. *J Neuropathol Exp Neurol,* 2009, 68(7): 709–735.

Meehan, W.P., III, R. Mannix, R. Zafonte. and A. Pascual-Leone. Chronic traumatic encephalopathy and athletes. *Neurology,* 2015, 85(17): 1504–1511.

Meehan, W.P., III, P. d'Hemecourt, and R.D. Comstock. High school concussions in the 2008–2009 academic year: Mechanism, symptoms, and management. *Am J Sports Med,* 2010, 38(12): 2405–2409.

Noy, S., S. Krawitz, and M.R. Del bigio. Chronic traumatic encephalopathy-like abnormalities in a routine neuropathology service. *J Neuropathol Exp Neurol,* 2016, 75(12): 1145–1154.

Omalu, B.I., et al. Chronic traumatic encephalopathy in a national football league player: Part II. *Neurosurgery,* 2006, 59(5): 1086–1092; discussion 1092–1093.

Omalu, B.I., et al. Chronic traumatic encephalopathy in a National Football League player. *Neurosurgery,* 2005, 57(1): 128–134; discussion 128–134.

Rothman, K.J. *Epidemiology: An Introduction.* Oxford: Oxford University Press, 2002.

Silverberg, N.D., et al. The nature and clinical significance of pre-injury recall bias following mild traumatic brain injury. *J Head Trauma Rehabil,* 2016, 31(6): 388–396.

13

PREVENTING LONG-TERM PROBLEMS: CONSIDERING WHETHER THE CUMULATIVE EFFECTS OF CONCUSSION CAN BE PREVENTED

Mark Savard's history of previous concussions was well known. In fact, he had already missed 23 games that season after sustaining his fifth documented concussion when on January 22, 2011, he was in Denver Colorado playing ice hockey for the Boston Bruins. It was the second period and the Colorado Avalanche were leading by a score of 2–1. Savard had just moved the puck behind and around the Avalanche's goal when Matt Hunwick, his former teammate, finished his check. Savard's head bounced off the Plexiglas. He immediately grabbed his head and fell to the ice. Savard himself, in subsequent interviews, reported that he was unable to see anything despite the fact that his eyes were open. Marc Savard had suffered his sixth and final sport-related concussion. He never played in the National Hockey League again.

As discussed in previous chapters, there is likely a cumulative effect of concussions; each sport-related concussion leaves an effect on the brain, albeit small, that likely never completely resolves. Therefore, many readers may be wondering whether athletes can decrease their risk of developing cumulative effects from multiple sport-related concussions.

Currently, the management of sport-related concussion involves removing the athlete from sport, ensuring that they decrease the risk of getting struck in the head again and thereby suffering an additional concussion prior to full recovery from the first. Recent experiments using animal models of concussion have shown some benefit to this. By spacing out repeated concussions over a longer period of time, the effects on learning and memory of animals that have sustained multiple concussions are diminished: the longer the time interval between injuries, the smaller the effect of repeated concussions on the ability to learn and remember. Therefore, the current practice of removing athletes from play until they are completely recovered and possibly adding in a longer symptom-free waiting period may be providing some long-term benefits if humans behave similarly to animals.

Clinical research has also shed some light on this. In a study of patients cared for in an emergency department who were diagnosed with a recent concussion, those athletes who had sustained previous concussions had higher symptom levels and took longer to recover from their recent injury than those who were there with their first injury. This suggests that there is a cumulative effect of concussion that shows up, at the very least, when another concussion is sustained. If, however, the previous concussion had occurred more than a year prior to the injury that brought them to the emergency department, there was little, if any, effect on overall symptom level or on the duration of symptoms. Those patients who had sustained a concussion within the previous year, however, had higher levels of symptoms when they presented to the emergency department and took longer to recover from their symptoms. This would suggest that there is a benefit to spacing out concussions over time; a concussion that occurs a year or more later than a prior injury has less of an effect, if any, than a concussion that has occurred within the year. Athletes benefit from waiting longer after injury before putting themselves at risk for additional concussions by returning to their sports.

Furthermore, as discussed in the previous chapter there is a and abnormal form of the protein tau known as *cis*-tau, which is associated with repetitive trauma to the head and thought to be the cause of some signs and symptoms. Repeating a mild concussion over and over again can result in the accumulation of this abnormal form of *cis*-tau in animal models. Moreover, if the animal is then left alive for several months, the *cis*-tau will spread by itself throughout the brain even in the absence of additional concussions. This would suggest that once the process of *cis*-tau formation has begun, it may carry on and spread throughout the brain even in the absence of additional trauma to the head. Two scientists mentioned previously, Drs. Lu and Zhou, have studied an antibody that was originally developed as a potential treatment for Alzheimer's disease. In animal studies, this antibody blocks the formation and spread of this abnormal *cis*-tau protein after repeated concussions. In addition, blocking this protein appears to spare some of the effects on behavior associated with it in the animal models. While preliminary, this research represents a potential future treatment for any potential cumulative effects associated with concussion and related to *cis*-tau. If indeed this abnormal form of tau is associated with signs and symptoms later in life, potentially they could be prevented or mitigated by administration of this antibody. It is still, however, in preliminary animal-based studies.

In addition, there is a drug that is sometimes used to treat Alzheimer's disease as well as dementia due to other causes. In preliminary animal studies of repeated concussions sustained by rodents, the administration of this drug diminishes the effects of repeated concussion to the cells of the brain as well as prevents some of the abnormal functioning that occurs after repeated concussions. Once again these studies are preliminary.

There are potential nonpharmacological treatments that may diminish any potential effects of repeated concussions on brain function and even on a cellular level. Both regular exercise and regular stimulation of the brain, particularly learning new skills, are associated with a decreased risk of cognitive impairment and a dementia later in life. When rodents that are subjected to repetitive concussions are housed in an enriched environment that allows for both physical as well as cognitive activity to a greater degree than the typical unenriched housing, the repetitive injuries they sustain have less of an effect on their motor skills, their behavior, and less effect on the cells of the brain than when they are housed in a normal, unenriched environment. This would suggest that regular exercise and regular stimulation of the brain may reduce any potential effects of repeated concussions. Once again, these studies are preliminary, but as there is little harm to regular exercise and cognitive stimulation and there are already known, well-established benefits of each, it seems prudent for all athletes to maintain a regular exercise regimen and a regular regimen of cognitive stimulation even after they retire from organized sports.

Furthermore, there are many other medical conditions that are associated with decreased cognitive function, headaches, depression, and other problems. These medical conditions include sleep apnea, obesity, depression, heart disease, physical inactivity, and several others. Optimizing the treatment of these medical conditions is important for all those suffering from them. If, however, repetitive concussions lead to similar long-term problems, then optimizing the treatment of these associated medical conditions is of particular importance to athletes who have sustained multiple concussions.

Lastly, while the focus of this chapter has been on concussions, there is a lot of discussion about whether subconcussive blows; those blows to the head that do not result in the signs and symptoms necessary for diagnosing a concussion may have cumulative effects later in life. This hypothesis has been proposed, since some athletes who have suffered from various problems later in life and some athletes who have been diagnosed postmortem with chronic traumatic encephalopathy (CTE) do not always have a history of formally diagnosed concussions. Thus, the hypothesis that subconcussive blows leads to these issues has been raised.

It is hard, however, to distinguish athletes who have suffered from concussions from those who have not. Recall that concussion is difficult to diagnose, especially without athletes regularly reporting their symptoms. As has been noted multiple times throughout this book, athletes are often reluctant to report their symptoms or do not recognize their symptoms as a concussion. This was particularly true in the past when the athletes included in many previous studies were playing their sports. Therefore, it could be that these athletes suffered multiple concussions but they were never formally diagnosed. To date, there is no reliable evidence that subconcussive blows lead to any long term problems.

In order to address the question as to whether there was an effect of subconcussive blows sustained during sports, a study of approximately 2,000 former collegiate athletes between the ages of 40 and 70 years was conducted by researchers at Boston Children's Hospital. In order to isolate any potential effect of subconcussive blows, as opposed to effects of concussion, those former athletes with a history of a diagnosed concussion were removed from analysis. The remaining athletes were separated into two groups: Those who participated in collision sports and those who participated in noncontact sports. Collision sports were defined as those sports during which body-to-body collisions occur routinely as a legal and expected part of the game. Those sports included football, rugby, men's ice hockey, and men's lacrosse. Noncontact sports were defined as those during which body to body contact was a rare and unexpected part of the game. Those sports included swimming, cross-country, golf, tennis, squash, Frisbee, and volleyball. Quality-of-life measures regarding cognitive function, mental health, sleep disturbance, and others were measured and compared between the two groups. There was no significant difference in the scores between collision sport athletes and non-contact sport athletes with one exception: collision sport athletes were more likely to suffer from negative consequences of alcohol use. While it is possible that this finding was a result of their exposure to collision sports, it is equally possible that those athletes who choose to participate in collision sports are also more likely to use alcohol frequently. Indeed, prior research at the college level suggested alcohol use is higher among team sport athletes than individual sport athletes. Since nearly all collision sports are team sports, and many of the noncontact sports including swimming, cross-country, golf, tennis, squash are individual sports, it may be that the frequency of alcohol use was different between these athletes even prior to their collegiate sports careers. The authors concluded that quality-of-life measures are similar between former collision sport athletes and former noncontact sport athletes with the possible exception of negative consequences from alcohol use.

In summary, available data suggest that repeated concussions can lead to long-term problems later in life. There is preliminary evidence that increasing the amount of time between repeated concussions may diminish long-term effects. In addition, there are medications and potential antibodies that in early preliminary studies show promise in reducing the potential cumulative effects of repeated concussions. Maximizing health through regular aerobic exercise and cognitive stimulation may also help diminish any potential effects of repeated concussions on cognition. There is no reliable evidence that repeated subconcussive blows to the head result in long-term problems. However, as there is no known benefit to repeated trauma to the brain during sports, efforts to limit blows to the brain during sports, either concussive or subconcussive, should continue.

SUGGESTED READINGS

Bailes, J.E., M.L. Dashnaw, A.L. Petraglia, and R.C. Turner. Cumulative effects of repetitive mild traumatic brain injury. *Prog Neurol Surg*, 2014, 28: 50–62.

Eisenberg, M., J.Andrea, W.P. Meehan, III, and R. Mannix. Time interval between concussions and symptom duration. *Pediatrics*, 2013, 132(1): 8–17.

"I still should be playing" By Stan Grossfeld. *Boston Globe*, November 16, 2016.

Kondo, A., et al. Antibody against early driver of neurodegeneration cis P-tau blocks brain injury and tauopathy. *Nature*, 2015, 523(7561): 431–436.

Liu, X., J. Qiu, S. Alcon, J. Hashim, W.P. Meehan, III, R. Mannix. Environmental enrichment mitigates deficits after repetitive mild TBI. *J Neurotrauma*, In press.

Mannix, R., W.P. Meehan, III, et al. Clinical correlates in an experimental model of repetitive mild brain injury. *Ann Neurol*, 2013, 74(1): 65–75.

McAllister, T., and M. McCrea. Long-term cognitive and neuropsychiatric consequences of repetitive concussions and head-impact exposure. *J Athl Train*, 2017, 52(3): 309–317.

Meehan, W.P., III, J. Zhang, R. Mannix, and M.J. Whalen. Increasing recovery time between injuries improves cognitive outcome after repeat mild concussions in mice. *Neurosurgery*, 2012, 71(4): 885–892.

Mei, Z., J. Qiu, S. Alcon, J. Hashim, A. Rotenberg, Y. Sun, W.P. Meehan, III, and R. Mannix. Memantine improves outcomes after repetitive traumatic brain injury. *Behav Brain Res*, In press.

Mouzon, B., H. Chaytow, G. Crynen, C. Bachmeier, J. Stewart, M. Mullan, W. Stewart, and F. Crawford. Repetitive mild traumatic brain injury and a mouse model produces learning and memory deficits accompanied by histological changes. *J Neurotrauma*, 2012, 29(18): 2761–2773.

14

THE FEMALE ATHLETE: ARE GIRLS AND BOYS DIFFERENT WHEN IT COMES TO CONCUSSION?

In January 2010, Australian snowboarder Torah Bright was considered a favorite to win the Olympic gold medal. With an inspiring performance in the 2006 Olympics, and countless other demonstrations of her ability since, Bright was favored over her two American opponents. Approximately two weeks before her bid for the Olympic gold, she was at the Winter X Games in Aspen, Colorado. During a routine training run, Bright accelerated up the side of the half pipe wall. Once airborne she completed a 540-degree turn, something she had done many times before without difficulty. This time, however, she lost control in the air. She cascaded down the wall. Her arms, rotating backward in an effort to help her regain her balance, were not in position to break her fall. The edge of her board landed first, catching on the down slope of the half pipe, and sending her body spinning. Her head snapped backward as her body landed, the back of it, striking the ground sharply. She brought her hands to her head almost immediately. She moved little until medical help arrived. With a shot at the Olympic gold medal only weeks away, she lay on the cold snow, stunned and nearly motionless.

Torah Bright was concussed.

While sport-related concussion is most commonly discussed as an injury to male athletes, it is a growing concern in the female athlete as well. It is likely that the focus on male athletes stems from their involvement in contact and collision sports. Historically, male athletes have played these sports in much greater numbers than female athletes. In the past, male athletes played much more aggressively than female athletes did. But this has changed decidedly over the last several decades. More and more female athletes are participating in contact and even collision sports, such as rugby.

Currently, over 211,000 women participate in sports sponsored by the National Collegiate Athletic Association. It is estimated that 3.3 million female athletes participate in high school sports. The number of women participating in contact sports, collision sports, and even combat sports is on the rise.

A study by Dr. Andrea Stracciolini and her colleagues showed a steady increase in participation in collegiate sports by female athletes from the 1960s until the early 2000s. In their study, about 10 percent of women who attended Division III colleges participated in collegiate sports in the 1960s, compared to just over 50 percent of those who attended college since 1998. The last several decades have seen the formation of women's leagues for collision sports such as American football and rugby, as well as combat sports such as boxing. Laila Ali, the daughter of former heavyweight champion Muhammad Ali, became famous in the last decade after becoming a professional boxer. Indeed, while I was attending Boston College in the 1990s, the women's rugby team won the national championship. Along with this increase in popularity has come more aggressive and even ferocious play in women's sports. This has led to increased recognition of sport-related concussions sustained by female athletes.

Still, there are some differences between male and female athletes with respect to concussion. With regards to the percentage of female athletes sustaining a concussion within a given sport, some medical evidence suggests that female athletes are at higher risk than their male counterparts. Some medical studies conducted in sports played by both female and male athletes suggest that women suffer higher rates of concussion. Multiple investigators have noted higher rates of concussion in women's soccer and basketball than in men's soccer and basketball, both at the high school and college levels.

Several possible reasons for this discrepancy exist. Some researchers believe that female athletes are simply more honest than male athletes, reporting their injury more frequently. Others argue that perhaps the difference is cultural. Male athletes are often taught that they should "tough it out" through an injury and report that nothing bothers them even when they are injured. Several medical studies have shown that female athletes report more symptoms after sustaining sport-related concussions than male athletes. Furthermore, they tend to rank their symptoms as more severe. They often complain of having symptoms for longer periods of time than their male counterparts. Some argue that these studies provide evidence of female athletes being more honest than male athletes. In addition, more recent research has suggested that women have a better understanding of the symptoms of sport-related concussion when compared to their male colleagues, at least among high school athletes. It may be, therefore, that when women experience symptoms of a concussion they're more likely to recognize the symptoms due to a concussion and therefore more likely to report it than male athletes. It is equally possible, however, that female athletes have worse symptoms and take longer to recover than male athletes. Men may be just as honest but are truly recovering more quickly. Thus far, no one has been able to tease out these two possibilities.

If it is true that women and girls are more likely to sustain concussions and to require longer recovery times than male athletes, it begs the question: why? There are several possible reasons why female athletes may be more likely to sustain concussions and may take longer to recover from concussions.

Some researchers argue that the difference is biological. As we have already learned earlier in this book, concussion is due to a rapid, rotational acceleration of the brain at the time of impact. We have also learned that by strengthening the neck muscles, athletes might reduce their risk of sustaining sport-related concussions. A medical study by athletic trainer Ryan Tierney and colleagues showed that female athletes have 49 percent less muscle strength and 30 percent less neck muscle girth than male athletes. Given their larger mass, larger muscle mass, and increased neck muscle strength, male athletes may be less likely to sustain sport-related concussions than female athletes competing in the same sport. Adding support to this hypothesis, a study in the *Journal of Primary Prevention* published in 2014 by Dawn Comstock and colleagues showed that neck strength was a significant predictor of concussion. Specifically, for every one-pound increase in the strength of the muscles of the neck, the odds of sustaining a concussion decreased by approximately 5 percent.

In addition, in girls' soccer in particular, some studies suggest that female soccer players are more likely to close their eyes when attempting to head the ball when compared to their male colleagues. The authors suggests that perhaps lack of visual awareness that arises when female soccer players close their eyes as they attempt to head the ball explains increased incidence of concussion among female players.

Some doctors and scientists have suggested that the different concentrations of hormones circulating in the blood may change the risks of sustaining a concussion and recovering from a concussion. In particular, it has been suggested that the female sex hormone, estrogen, may make females more susceptible to concussive brain injury. The exact role of estrogen, however, is controversial. In laboratory experiments using rodents, giving estrogen to male mice has improved their outcome after a traumatic brain injury. Female rodents given extra estrogen prior to traumatic brain injuries, however, did markedly worse. Thus, the true effect of estrogen, if any, on outcome after traumatic brain injury remains unclear. Whether estrogen has any effect on the risk of sustaining a sport-related concussion or the recovery after suffering a sport-related concussion is unknown.

One of the advantages of computerized neuropsychological testing is that it allows us to measure or quantify the degree of injury, the degree of brain dysfunction after a concussion. Studies have revealed differences in cognitive function between male and female athletes. These differences are true both before and after injury. Clearly there are some differences in the way the brain operates between male and female athletes. In one study, collegiate women's soccer players who sustained a concussion had slower reaction times than male collegiate soccer players who sustained a concussion. Other studies have shown differences in memory between male and female athletes. Still, the role that these potential differences in cognitive function has on risk of sustaining a concussion or time required to recover from a concussion remains unknown.

In summary, there does appear to be differences in the risk of concussion between male and female athletes, with women and girls being at higher risk of sustaining injury. Similarly, there is some evidence suggesting that female athletes might take longer to recover from concussions than male athletes. The reasons for these potential discrepancies are unknown. Honesty in reporting, differences in muscle mass or strength, varying hormone levels, or discrepancies in cognitive abilities are all being considered as potential factors.

SUGGESTED READINGS

Broshek, D.K., et al. Sex differences in outcome following sports-related concussion. *J Neurosurg*, 2005, 102(5): 856–863.

Clark, J.F., H.T. Elgendy-Peerman, J.G. Divine, R.E. Mangine, K.A. Hasselfeld, J.C. Khoury, and A.J. Colosimo. Lack of eye discipline during headers in high school girls soccer: A possible mechanism for increased concussion rates. *Med Hypotheses*, 2017, 100: 10–14.

Collins, C.L., E.N. Fletcher, S.K. Fields, L. Kluchurosky, M.K. Rohrkemper, R.D. Comstock, and R.C. Cantu. Neck strength: A protective factor reducing risk for concussion in high school sports. *J Prim Prev*, 2014, 35(5): 309–319.

Colvin, A.C., et al. The role of concussion history and gender in recovery from soccer-related concussion. *Am J Sports Med*, 2009, 37(9): 1699–1704.

Covassin, T., C.B. Swanik, and M.L. Sachs. Sex differences and the incidence of concussions among collegiate athletes. *J Athl Train*, 2003, 38(3): 238–244.

Covassin, T., et al. Sex differences in baseline neuropsychological function and concussion symptoms of collegiate athletes. *Br J Sports Med*, 2006, 40(11): 923–927; discussion 927.

Covassin, T., P. Schatz, and C.B. Swanik. Sex differences in neuropsychological function and post-concussion symptoms of concussed collegiate athletes. *Neurosurgery*, 2007, 61(2): 345–350; discussion 350–351.

Farace, E. and W.M. Alves. Do women fare worse? A metaanalysis of gender differences in outcome after traumatic brain injury. *Neurosurg Focus*, 2000, 8(1): e6.

Gessel, L.M., et al. Concussions among United States high school and collegiate athletes. *J Athl Train*, 2007, 42(4): 495–503.

Khodaee, M., D.W. Currie, I.M. Asif, and R.D. Comstock. Nine-year study of US high school soccer injuries: Data from a national sports injury surveillance programme. *Br J Sports Med*, December 28, 2016 [Epub ahead of print].

Thomas, D.J., K. Coxe, H. Li, T.L. Pommering, J.A. Young, G.A. Smith, and J. Yang. Length of recovery from sports-related concussions in pediatric patients treated at concussion clinics. *Clin J Sport Med*, January 12, 2017 [Epub ahead of print].

Tierney, R.T., et al. Gender differences in head-neck segment dynamic stabilization during head acceleration. *Med Sci Sports Exerc*, 2005, 37(2): 272–279.

Wallace, J., et al. Sex differences in high school athletes knowledge of sport-related concussion symptoms and reporting behaviors. *J Athl Train*, 2017 [Epub ahead of print].

15

Setting Up a Concussion Program

On Friday September 25, 2009, talk show host Conan O'Brien was engaged in a mini mock triathlon against *Desperate Housewives* star Teri Hatcher. The last leg of the event consisted of a footrace. As they descended the studio stairs, Hatcher had a slight lead. They mounted the stage and dashed for the finish line. Approximately 6 feet before the finish line, O'Brien's legs slid out in front of him. He fell backwards. The back of his head struck the ground with an audible "boom." Per his own report on a later show, O'Brien had confusion for several minutes after the event. He said, "In the moment, I saw stars. But I tried to keep going." He was unable to recall the year. He was unfamiliar with his remaining duties for the show. He had significant amnesia for the events following the injury.

Conan O'Brien was concussed.

That's right. Concussion doesn't only happen during organized sports. Those of us in the field of sports medicine must be prepared to care for our athletes' injuries, regardless of where or how they occur. A comprehensive concussion program will help in that effort.

Many readers will recall that in the 1980s concussion was not considered a serious injury. It is only during that decade that medical investigators started examining the effects of concussion on brain function. Much of the medical and scientific evidence reviewed in this book is relatively new. The current approaches to assessing and managing concussive brain injury are also relatively new. Many medical professionals will be unaware of some of these findings, guidelines, and recommendations. This should not be alarming. Medical information does not come about as the result of one or two studies. Medical practice changes only as a result of many studies, investigating various aspects of a medical problem, and all pointing to a similar conclusion. Given the other injuries, illnesses, and diseases that medical professionals must manage, concussion may represent a very small proportion of an individual clinician's practice. Therefore, the first step in setting up a comprehensive concussion management program will be to identify a clinician who is well-versed and knowledgeable about the assessment and management of sport-related concussions. In many communities, such an individual may not be readily available. In this case, clinicians who are interested in the assessment and management of concussive brain injuries should be encouraged to review the available medical literature and start a management program from scratch.

Given the persistent increase in media attention paid toward a sport-related concussion and concussive injury of the brain in general, it should be easier at the time of publication of this addition to identify a concussion expert in your area than it was at the time of the first addition. Still, in more rural settings where there are fewer medical professionals, other pressing issues in medicine will likely take precedent over sport-related concussion and concussive brain injury. Therefore, it still may be difficult to find an expert in the area. For clinicians who are interested in becoming an expert in this area, there are many conferences, text books, and online tutorials designed for medical professionals interested in learning more about this injury, and its diagnosis, assessment, and management.

Ideally, a comprehensive concussion management program consists of many medical professionals from different specialties as opposed to a single clinician. Ideal programs include athletic trainers, physicians, neuropsychologists, other medical clinicians such as nurse practitioners or physician assistants, sports psychologists, and physical therapists. The roles of each of these medical professionals will be discussed in further detail below.

Once clinicians have been identified who will assess and manage the sport-related concussions of a given group of athletes, they must decide collectively which standardized assessments will be used. A standard symptom inventory should be used among all clinicians for all athletes. Likewise, a standard balance assessment should be used by all clinicians and for all at risk athletes. The balance assessment should be measured and scored in precisely the same way by all individuals participating in the program. This will allow for consistent measurements. Similarly, a single standardized sideline concussion assessment tool should be chosen so that all clinicians are performing the same sideline assessment on every athlete. Finally, a computerized neurocognitive assessment should be chosen and a baseline assessment should be performed on every at risk athlete.

As mentioned previously there are several different symptom inventories available. Prior to the start of the season the clinicians who will be caring for the athletes should get together and decide which symptom inventory they will use. They must decide whether, during the baseline assessment, an athlete should score any particular symptom he or she is experiencing on the day of the baseline assessment, or whether all athletes who are not currently concussed at the time of the baseline assessment should score a zero. Therefore, after injury athletes would only score those symptoms that resulted from the concussion. For readers who are looking to start a comprehensive concussion management plan but are unfamiliar with symptom inventories, the standardized concussion assessment tool version 5 (SCAT 5) is available for free online and includes an excellent symptom inventory known as the post-concussion symptoms scale. At the time of this writing, typing "SCAT 5" into the Google search bar and clicking on the third recommended link will take you to a free, downloadable version of the SCAT 5.

Baseline balance assessment must also be obtained for every athlete prior to the start of the season. There are several versions of the balance error scoring system available. Perhaps the easiest to use and most accessible to the reader is the modified balance error scoring system (mBESS) proposed as part of the SCAT 5. Again, it is available for free online.

They must also decide on which sideline assessment they will use. This decision should be made primarily by the clinician who will be on the side of the field, ice rink, or court and is most likely to be present when a concussion occurs. For most athletic teams, this will be the athletic trainer. Again, several sideline concussion assessments are available and have been reviewed previously in this book. Some are available for free online, including those associated with the SCAT 5.

Finally, the group must decide which computerized neurocognitive assessment, if any, will be used. This will depend heavily on which clinicians will be caring for the athletes. Each of the computerized neurocognitive assessments uses different testing paradigms, different ways of scoring the test, and different ways of reporting athletes' scores. The clinicians, regardless of their background, need to undertake training in the specific computerized neurocognitive assessment chosen in order to correctly administer and interpret these tests. There are several versions available. Readers who are starting a comprehensive concussion management program in the area should contact a local physician or neuropsychologist experienced in the assessment and management of sport-related concussions in order to determine which computerized neurocognitive assessment will be best for their program. If no such clinician is available in your area, athletic trainers can often be useful in identifying a doctor or other clinician who might be interested in collaborating in a comprehensive concussion management program.

In most cases, the athletic trainer will coordinate the baseline assessments of the athletes, ensuring that a baseline symptom inventory, a baseline balance assessment, a baseline sideline assessment, and a baseline computerized neurocognitive test is obtained for every athlete. As the athletic trainer will often be on the sidelines, courtside or rink side when the concussion occurs, it is the athletic trainer who will be responsible for repeating the sideline assessment when diagnosing an athlete with a sport-related concussion. The athletic trainer will ensure that the athlete is not returned to sport until completely recovered from the concussion. The athletic trainer will coordinate all required follow-up and medical appointments.

The team physician's presence can vary based on availability, team resources, and other factors. Ideally, the team physician is present at all competitions. For many teams, the athletic trainer will respond first to all injuries. The team physician will be available to the athletic trainer for any injury that requires further medical assessment. In other settings, the athletic trainer and team physician will respond to injury simultaneously. In some circumstances, the team physician may not be present at competitions. In these situations the team physician's role is to see the athletes in clinic, provide further assessment, treatment, and coordinate all out-patient care. In an ideal program, the athletic trainer and team physician work closely together.

Nurse practitioners and physician assistants function similarly to the team physician, and usually under the guidance or supervision of the team physician. While in some cases they may be present at athletic events, their main role is in the clinic where they will assess and manage injuries on an outpatient basis.

Many teams may have a designated neuropsychologist who works closely with the team physician in the assessment and management of sport-related concussions. Neuropsychologists will help make the diagnosis of the sport-related concussion, particularly in situations where the diagnosis may be somewhat unclear. They may administer and interpret both computerized neuropsychological tests as well as traditional neuropsychological tests in order to ascertain an athlete's brain function. They will prescribe therapies and strategies to help an athlete recover from his or her concussion. They will provide academic accommodations for student athletes, which allow athletes to safely participate in school while recovering from their concussions. They will help determine when an athlete has recovered from his or her concussion. They will guide the athlete in safely returning to play.

As noted previously, while most athletes will recover from their concussions relatively quickly, a minority of athletes will take several weeks to months to recover completely from their sport-related concussions. Such prolonged recoveries can often have negative effects on an athlete's mood, behavior, and overall disposition. In these circumstances, a sports psychologist, or, if a sports psychologist is unavailable, a general psychologist, will be useful in counseling, teaching coping strategies, and assessing for more serious mood disorders. While few teams will have a dedicated sports psychologist, most team physicians will have a sports psychologist with whom they work closely and may refer athletes in need.

The physical therapist in most concussion programs will be used to prepare an athlete who sustains a sport-related concussion for a safe return to sports. As noted previously, once the athlete is recovered he or she should not be returned directly into competition, especially after a period of prolonged rest. After long periods of rests, athletes become weaker, slower. They lose some of their agility and confidence. Their strength, conditioning, speed, reaction time, and confidence, all need to be restored prior to returning to competition. Therefore, athletes who have recently recovered from a concussion will start by engaging in some light aerobic activity. They will advance along several return-to-play stages in a stepwise fashion, advancing to more rigorous forms of exercise only if they remain symptom-free at previous levels. Physical therapists can help monitor this return to play. They can ensure that prior to returning to competition an athlete is fast, agile, strong. Returning to play prior to achieving adequate speed, agility, and strength places an athlete at increased risk for any sport-related injury, not only concussion. Therefore, these important phases of return to play should not be ignored. Standard return to play stages, from the Fifth International Conference on Concussion in Sports, are shown in Table 15.1.

Given the body of literature that has come out since publication of the first addition of this book showing that an earlier return to a sub-symptom threshold level of physical activity is beneficial, there is a new roll to be play by physical therapists. Physical therapists can be useful in monitoring exercise levels in an athlete who is currently recovering from a sport-related concussion. Furthermore, many athletes suffer from vestibular symptoms after a concussion. There is a sub-certification of physical therapy known as vestibular therapy. Vestibular therapists can be useful in helping alleviate some of the symptoms of the vestibular system that can occur after a concussion. In addition to vestibular symptoms, there is building evidence that suggests normal oculomotor function, the movement of the eyes, can be disrupted after a concussion.

Table 15.1
Graduated Return-to-Sport Strategy

Stage	Aim	Activity	Goal of Each Step
1	Symptom limited activity	Daily activities that do not provoke symptoms	Gradual reintroduction of work/school activities
2	Light aerobic exercise	Walking or stationary cycling at slow to medium pace. No resistance training	Increased heart rate
3	Sport-specific exercise	Running or skating drills. No head impact activities	Add movement
4	Non-contact training drills	Harder training drills, e.g., passing drills. It may start progressive resistance training	Exercise, coordination and increased thinking
5	Full contact practice	Following medical clearance, participate in normal training activities	Restore confidence and assess functional skills by coaching staff
6	Return to sport	Normal game play	

NOTE: An initial period of 24–48 hours of both relative physical rest and cognitive rest is recommended before beginning the RTS progression. There should be at least 24 hours (or longer) for each step of the progression. If any symptoms worsen during exercise, the athlete should go back to the previous step. Resistance training should be added only in the later stages (stage 3 or 4 at the earliest). If symptoms are persistent (e.g., more than 10–14 days in adults or more than 1 month in children), the athlete should be referred to a health care professional who is an expert in the management of concussion.

Source: Adapted from McCrory, P., et al. "Consensus statement on concussion in sport: The Fifth International Conference on Concussion in Sport held in Berlin, October 2016." *Br J Sports Med.* Published Online First: April 26, 2017. doi: 10.1136/bjsports-2017-097699.

Seeing an optometrist to have a proper evaluation can lead to exercises that will help restore normal visual and ocular function. Therefore, knowing an optometrist that specializes in oculomotor dysfunction after traumatic brain injury would be helpful in order to refer athletes when needed.

Once all personnel have been identified, have agreed to participate, and have been appropriately trained in assessing and managing sport-related concussions, baseline assessments should be made and the concussion management team should meet and discuss a plan of action. The plan of action should include which preseason baseline assessments will be performed, who will perform them, and when they will be performed. The plan should include guidelines for the acute response to injury, for the clinical, outpatient management, and for return-to-play. The following is an example of a concussion action plan. These plans of action are most effective if written down and distributed to all medical personnel, coaches, parents, and other people involved with the team.

A concussion action plan, or concussion protocol, is a written document developed by all members of the sports medicine team. It consists of seven major components.

I. The definition of concussion. The concussion action plan often starts by defining concussive brain injury and describing some of the characteristics of a concussion, including some of the ways athletes sustain concussions.

II. The signs and symptoms of concussion. Often, the concussion action plan will contain lists or tables that review for the sports medical team the signs and symptoms most often associated with sport-related concussions.

III. Preseason items. All actions that should be performed prior to the start of the season are described in this section of the concussion action plan. The baseline assessments that the sports medicine team has chosen to obtain on all at risk athletes will be described in this section. Any cervical muscle strengthening or other preventative strategies will also be included here.

IV. On-site response to injury. This section details the immediate response to an injured athlete. It should review proper techniques for immobilizing an athlete and transporting an athlete to a local emergency department when necessary. For athletes who sustain less emergent injuries, specifics are given for monitoring the athlete after injury. Often this section will include instructions to be given to the athlete, the athlete's roommates or family members, and others who will be with the athlete for the 24 hours following the injury.

V. Out-patient response to injury. This section describes how the athlete will be managed during the days and weeks following a sport-related concussion. It will describe which providers are involved in the care of the concussed athlete. It will describe some initial therapies as well as which members of the larger team or school community need to be notified. Concussion action plans at academic institutions will often include academic planning and how academic accommodations can be put into place for the concussed athlete. Which members of the sports medicine team will discuss the situation with school administrators is often discussed in this section. Usually, this part of the concussion action plan includes the requirements for determining when an athlete has completely recovered from his or her concussion.

VI. Off-campus injuries. Although it is most common for athletes to sustain their concussions while participating in sports, concussions also occur outside of sports. The truly detailed concussion action plan includes an approach to assessing and treating those concussions that occur outside of organized sports activity.

VII. Return to play. Specific guidelines for returning an athlete to play who has recently recovered from a sport-related concussion are discussed. The stages that must precede the return to game play, the monitoring of the stages, and the specific activities allowed during each stage are often outlined in this section. In addition, given the changes in the most recent consensus summary and agreement statement from the International Conference on Concussion in Sport, this section might include the types of light aerobic activity that could be initiated after the first few days of a concussion and ways to maintain them at a sub-symptom threshold level.

Not all concussion action plans are the same. Not all contain every section listed. Others may contain information not mentioned here. The action plan should be tailored to suit the needs of the athletes covered by it. It should be adjusted to account for the circumstances, sports being played, type of sports equipment being worn, playing surfaces, number of personnel involved, type of personnel involved, and available resources. In order to give the reader an idea of what a concussion action plan looks like, one is included in the Appendix. It is based on the concussion protocol used at Boston College in Chestnut Hill, Massachusetts. This is one of the best concussion protocols I have come across. Some of the terms are in medical jargon, and you may not be familiar with their meaning. In addition, the resources available to the sports medicine team at Boston College are much greater than they will be for many providers involved at the high school, use, and other levels. Furthermore, as with all protocols, this will be adjusted as new findings with regards to sport-related concussion and its treatment are discovered. Therefore, this template is meant to be used simply as a template that offers some framework that for medical personnel involved in your concussion protocol to use when designing their own protocol. These medical personnel will be familiar with these terms and aware of what resources will be available to them. In addition, several of the appendices noted in this sample concussion action plan are included elsewhere in this book, and therefore, not duplicated in the Appendix.

In summary, the ideal concussion program involves many clinicians in various specialties, all working together to care for concussed athletes. The best concussion management plans start before the athlete ever takes to the field, court, or ice, by obtaining baseline measurements. Identifying medical providers with an interest in managing athletes who sustain concussions is the first step in trying to organize a concussion management program. For clinicians working with a given team, school, or other group of athletes, a written concussion action plan can help ensure that athletes receive the best possible care.

Suggested Readings

Lovell, M.R., R. J. Echemendia, J.T. Barth, and M.W. Collins. *Traumatic Brain Injury in Sports: An International Neuropsychological Perspective.* Lisse, The Netherlands: Swets and Zeitlinger, 2004.

McCrea, M. *Mild Traumatic Brain Injury and Postconcussion Syndrome: The New Evidence Base for Diagnosis and Treatment.* New York: Oxford University Press, 2008.

McCrory, P., et al. Consensus statement on concussion in sport: The Fifth International Conference on Concussion in Sport held in Berlin, October 2016. *Br J Sports Med,* April 26, 2017 [Epub ahead of print].

16

THE FUTURE: WHAT MEDICAL RESEARCH MAY LEAD TO IN THE FUTURE

On August 11, 2005, New York Mets were playing the San Diego Padres. The score was tied at one run each when a pop fly was hit between right field and center field. The center fielder, Carlos Beltran, started sprinting for the ball as did the right fielder, Mike Cameron. Both men were going full speed when they dove for the ball. They struck each other head-to-head. Each man was knocked unconscious. Both men were concussed. Cameron also suffered facial bone fractures to the nose and cheek bone.

When it comes to athletes sustaining concussions in sports, many unanswered questions remain:

1. Is there a genetic predisposition to concussion and can athletes be tested for it?
2. Is there a medication that might effectively treat concussive brain injury, as opposed to only treating the symptoms?
3. Is there a medication that can prevent the cumulative effects of concussions?
4. Is exercise helpful during recovery from concussion?
5. Do the restrictions on activities often recommended after a concussion result in symptoms of their own that might be attributed to a concussion?
6. Do repetitive concussions cause chronic traumatic encephalopathy (CTE)? Do subconcussive blows?
7. Is there a potential treatment for CTE?
8. Are there risk factors besides trauma to the brain that can result in CTE?
9. Is there a blood test or other objective measure that that might be used to determine when an athlete has sustained a concussion or when an athlete has completely recovered from a concussion?
10. Is there a type of imaging that can allow doctors to "see" a concussion?

Future medical and scientific research will seek to answer these questions. These efforts will likely focus on:

- Discovering more about what happens to the brain when an athlete is concussed.
- Discovering whether certain athletes are predisposed to sustaining concussions or predisposed to bad outcomes after sustaining multiple sport-related concussions.

- Discovering how we can more accurately diagnose a sport-related concussion, determining when athletes' symptoms are attributable to concussions from which they are incompletely recovered and when they are attributable to other reasons.
- Determining precisely when the athlete has recovered completely from his or her sport-related concussion.
- Discovering potential treatments that will assist athletes in recovering from sport-related concussions, helping them recover faster, and helping them prevent any long-term problems.
- Discovering treatments that may prevent or otherwise mitigate the cumulative effects from concussion.
- Discovering treatments and preventative measures for CTE.

Some of the most recent medical studies are discussed here.

ACCELEROMETERS

One of the newest technologies used to investigate sport-related concussions uses a device known as an accelerometer. Accelerometers are small sensors that are placed into the helmets of athletes during practice or competition. These sensors can be used to measure the amount of force of a given impact. They can measure the speed and direction a helmet moves after impact. They record how fast and in what direction the helmet spins after an impact. These measurements can then be correlated to athletes who sustain a sport-related concussion. The characteristics of the impacts causing sport-related concussions can be compared to those impacts that do not result in a sport-related concussion. These data might help us understand more about what exactly it is that leads to concussive brain injury.

Preliminary data using these sensors have revealed that concussion occur after a wide range of forces, resulting in a wide range of accelerations. Symptoms do not necessarily correlate with the amount of force involved in the impact, or with the maximum acceleration produced by the impact. This suggests that other factors play a significant part in determining whether a concussion occurs or not and how long it takes to recover from a concussion.

PREDISPOSITION

Some athletes may be predisposed to concussion, meaning they may be more likely to suffer a sport-related concussion than other athletes. Similarly, some athletes, while they may not be more likely to sustain sport-related concussions, may be more vulnerable to the effects of concussions. They may be more likely than other athletes to suffer long-term problems after sustaining multiple concussions. They may suffer more diminished cognitive function after sustaining concussions. They may suffer from longer recovery times than other athletes. The ability to identify these athletes could be used to prevent injuries.

For example, if there was a test that could determine which athletes are more likely to sustain sport-related concussions, athletes could be screened prior to participating in high-risk sports. Those who tested positive, and therefore knew that they were more vulnerable to sustaining a sport-related concussion, might choose to participate in safer sports, such as swimming, rather than higher-risk sports such as football and ice hockey. Another option would be to test only those athletes who had sustained at least one sport-related concussion. Those who after sustaining their first sport-related concussion were found to be at increased risk compared to other athletes might choose not to play high-risk sports. Those who underwent the test and were not found to be at increased risk of sustaining sport-related concussions might choose to continue playing.

Similarly, if physicians could predict which athletes were more likely to suffer a bad outcome after sustaining a sport-related concussion or multiple concussions, they could use this information to help athletes decide whether to continue playing high-risk contact or collision sports or not. Efforts have been made to identify just such a test.

Some medical studies indicate that certain athletes may have a genetic predisposition to poor outcome after sustaining a concussion, multiple concussions, or even multiple repeated blows to the head that do not cause concussions. The most well-studied gene is known as apolipoprotein E epsilon 4, or *APOE4* for short. Some of the earliest medical literature to study *APOE4* was performed in boxers. A physician named Barry Jordan assessed neurological status of multiple retired boxers. He noted that those who carried this particular gene, *APOE4*, had worse brain function than those who did not. Boxers who had fought in more bouts and were therefore exposed to a greater number of blows to the head had worse brain function than those boxers who fought in fewer bouts over their careers. Those boxers who carried the *APOE4* gene *and* fought in a high number of bouts had the worst brain function.

Other medical studies, conducted outside of the realm of athletics, suggest that people who carry this particular gene and who also sustain a concussion or other traumatic brain injury at some point during their lifetime are at increased risk of poor outcomes, including an increased risk of Alzheimer's disease.

These studies are preliminary, however. The effects of carrying *APOE4* on neurological function after brain injury are poorly understood. Some studies show that *APOE4* has no effect on outcome after sustaining a head injury. In fact, in some patients, having the *APOE4* gene may be beneficial. *APOE4* may be beneficial for children who sustain an injury to the brain. Combined, these studies suggest that the effects of *APOE4* after a traumatic brain injury may be different depending on how old a person is at the time of injury.

In order to help further understand the role age may play in determining the effects of *APOE4* after traumatic brain injury, investigators have taken to the laboratory. One of my colleagues, Rebekah Mannix, MD, conducted an experiment in mice, which was published in the *Journal of Cerebral Blood Flow and Metabolism*. Some of the mice had the *APOE4* gene, and others did not. All mice underwent a traumatic brain injury. Adult mice that had the *APOE4* gene had worse brain function after injury than mice without the *APOE4* gene. However, immature or "pediatric" mice with the *APOE4* gene had the same brain function after injury as mice without the *APOE4* gene. Her results suggest that the *APOE4* may have harmful effects for adult mice who sustain a traumatic brain injury, while in pediatric mice that sustain a traumatic brain injury, *APOE4* may have no effect. Experiments continue to try and determine exactly what APOE does after brain injury that seems to affect the outcome and why the effects seem to be different based on the age at the time of injury.

These experiments are exciting. They offer hope, that one day we may be able to predict which athletes are at risk for poor outcomes after a concussion. **However, until we learn more about APOE, its function after brain injury, whether the results are consistent, and how age affects outcome, it cannot be used clinically to treat athletes. Currently, APOE 4 is not a useful test, and should not be measured in patients, athletes or otherwise, for the purpose of trying to assess outcome after traumatic brain injury.**

MARKERS OF INJURY

In addition to genes, researchers have also searched for blood tests that might be associated with concussive brain injury, brain function after injury, and perhaps, be used to monitor recovery from injury. "Serum markers" are proteins, chemicals, or other molecules in the blood that can be used to identify a certain disease or disease process. Two of the most commonly discussed serum markers that have been investigated for the assessment of concussive brain injury are the "S-100B" protein and "neuron specific enolase" (NSE). In a study out of Germany published in 2001 in the *Journal of Neurology, Neurosurgery and Psychiatry*, Herrmann and colleagues measured S-100B and NSE in patients who had sustained traumatic brain injuries, mostly concussions. Both serum markers, S-100b and NSE, were measured on the first, second, and third days after injury. Patients had their brain function measured two weeks after admission to the hospital and again six months later. Those patients who had more S-100B and NSE in their blood after injury had worse brain function, both in the tests performed soon after injury and those performed six months later. These finding suggest that these two serum markers might prove useful in determining which athletes will suffer significant and prolonged losses of brain function after concussion. Other studies have also found that theses serum markers may be useful in identifying patients who have sustained a traumatic brain injury or in identifying those at risk for prolonged recovery after injury.

However, these findings have not been consistent. Some studies have failed to reveal any utility in testing for S-100B or NSE. Some studies show elevations in these serum markers in patients without brain injury. This suggests that there may be other reasons why these markers are elevated. Until further research has been conducted, neither of these serum markers can be used clinically, to assess and treat patients, with reliability. Other factors, besides genes and proteins in the blood, have also been studied. Many proteins can also be found in the urine and saliva. As neither urine nor saliva requires a needle stick in order to obtain a sample, these body fluids would likely be preferable to blood as a marker for concussion.

Researchers have investigated whether athletes who experience certain symptoms after their concussion have larger deficits in brain function or take longer to recover. A study performed at the University of Pittsburgh by neuropsychologist Micky Collins that was published in the *American Journal of Sports Medicine* in 2003, separated athletes who sustained a concussion into two groups: (1) those reporting a headache one week after their injury and (2) those without a headache. Their results showed that those athletes still reporting a headache one week after injury had worse memory and slower reaction times than those athletes not reporting a headache. The study also found that athletes reporting headaches were more likely to have suffered amnesia at the time of their injury. An additional study by many of the same investigators showed that athletes who suffered migraine headache symptoms after their concussions took longer to recover from their injuries than those athletes who did not report migraine headache-type symptoms.

This correlation between headaches and migraine headaches in particular and recovery from concussion led some researchers to wonder whether athletes who have suffered from migraine headaches in the past might be at increased risk of sustaining a concussion. Indeed, a study out of Canada, published in the *British Journal of Sports Medicine* in 2006, analyzed data collected by the Canadian Community Health Survey. Those athletes who were diagnosed as having migraine headaches by a health professional were more likely to have sustained a sport-related concussion in the previous 12 months than those athletes not diagnosed with migraines.

Headaches and migraines symptoms in particular are not the only symptoms being investigated as possible determinants of sport-related concussion recovery. After sustaining a concussion, many athletes will complain of feeling "in a fog." This is a subjective symptom, meaning it can be easily measured or quantified. Although many athletes use this term and have an inherent understanding of its meaning, it is difficult to define. Still, several clinicians have observed associations between this symptom, "fogginess," and poor outcome after sport-related concussion. A study published in the *Journal of the International*

Neuropsychological Society in 2004 measured overall concussion symptoms and neuropsychological test scores of athletes who reported feeling foggy and compared the findings to athletes who did not report feeling foggy. Athletes who reported fogginess experienced a larger number of other post-concussion symptoms than those not reporting fogginess. Furthermore, athletes who reported feeling foggy had slower reaction times, worse memory, and took more time to complete neurocognitive tasks than athletes not reporting fogginess.

Many other factors are being considered as potentially increasing an athlete's risk of either sustaining a concussion, suffering a long recovery after a concussion, or suffering long-term effects later in life after sustaining a concussion, or multiple concussions, earlier in life. Other illnesses or diseases such as attention deficit hyperactivity disorder, post-traumatic stress disorder, anxiety, and depression are all being investigated currently. Perhaps athletes on certain medications at the time of their injury may protect against the effects of concussion or worsen the outcome after concussion. The shape of the skull, musculature of the neck and shoulders, or other anatomic considerations may affect one's risk of concussion or recovery from concussion. Studies to look for these potential risk factors will hopefully lead to a better understanding of which athletes are at greatest risk.

IMAGING

Earlier in this book, we learned that pictures of the brain, such as computed tomograms of the head (head CTs) or magnetic resonance images (MRIs) appear normal in athletes who have sustained concussions. But there are other types of pictures available. Some investigators seek to discover ways of picturing or imaging the brain that can allow us to "see" a concussion in an injured athlete. Several such methods of imaging have been studied.

Functional MRI

Functional MRI (fMRI) is somewhat complicated to explain. Perhaps the easiest way to think about it is as a picture of the brain that allows doctors to see which parts of the brain are in use, receiving increased amounts of blood flow, while the patient is completing certain tasks. In other words, an athlete who is undergoing an fMRI after a concussion is asked to complete certain mathematical tasks. While the athlete completes these tasks, images or pictures are taken of the brain. These pictures have various parts of the brain lit up in different colors, based on how vigorously that part of the brain is being used and how much blood flow that part of the brain is receiving. It allows doctors to see which part of the brain is "activated" and how hard a given part of the brain is working.

Studies have shown that athletes who have sustained sport-related concussions use different parts of the brain to a higher degree than athletes who are not concussed. In addition, as athletes recover from their concussions, and regain their previous levels of brain functioning, the changes in their fMRIs go away. Once recovered, their fMRIs look similar to those of athletes who have not sustained a concussion.

Diffusion Tensor Imaging

Diffusion tensor imaging (DTI) is another variation on traditional MRI scanning. Again, DTI can be somewhat difficult to understand for readers without scientific or medical training. Perhaps the easiest way to think about it is as a picture or image of the brain that allows doctors to see the movement of water in the brain. Recall earlier in the book when we discussed the cells of the brain known as neurons. Each neuron had a long, narrow section known as the axon. Well, water inside of a neuron can travel down the length of the axon. But it can also travel perpendicular to the axon, across the cell membrane. Doctors can detect certain changes in the brain cells by measuring the direction in which the water of the brain is traveling. Studies in children and adolescents after concussive brain injury have shown abnormal DTIs of the brain, even though CT scans and traditional MRIs appear normal. Thus, DTI may help diagnose a concussion, even though the more traditional forms of brain imaging show normal results.

TREATMENTS

Currently, there are no known effective treatments for concussive brain injury. Physicians provide "supportive care" for patients with major concussive injuries. These patients are often comatose, or have such pronounced brain dysfunction that they cannot think clearly. "Supportive care" means that doctors help the patients breathe, maintain blood pressure, relieve pressure build-up in the brain due to swelling or bleeding, provide nutrition, and basically keep patients alive until they are able to recover from the injury on their own.

For patients with milder injury, as is more common for athletes, we can treat some of the symptoms of concussion. Therapies like the brief periods of physical and cognitive rest discussed previously, help to treat many of the symptoms. Academic accommodations can be used to help athletes obtain cognitive rest while in school. Some medications can be used to treat headaches, insomnia, poor cognitive function and other specific symptoms of concussion. But ultimately, there is no direct treatment for the concussion itself, no treatment that helps athletes recover faster. Discovering such a treatment is the main goal of many of us currently caring for athletes with concussions.

There are several potential options.

Three years ago, I attended a lecture given by Michael Whalen, MD. Dr. Whalen is the head of a laboratory in the neuroscience center of the

Massachusetts General Hospital that investigates traumatic brain injury. I approached him about developing a model of concussion which would allow us to study potential therapies. Since that time, we have developed models of severe, moderate and mild concussive brain injuries. These models can now be used to test potential treatments. In fact, by using these models, we have found a molecule that spares the loss of cognitive function after traumatic brain injury.

In addition, experiments performed in the laboratory of Rebekah Mannix, MD, at Boston Children's Hospital have shown the benefits of a medication that appears to improve the cellular changes that occur to the brains of mice subjected to repeated concussions. It also seems to improve some, but not all, aspects of function. As this medication seems to mitigate the accumulation of hyperphosphorylated tau in the brains of mice subjected to repeated concussion, it might represent a potential future treatment for CTE if hyperphosphorylated tau is in fact the agent causing symptoms experienced by those ultimately diagnosed with CTE.

Perhaps more strikingly, doctors Lu and Zhou at the Beth Israel Deaconess Medical Center in Boston have developed an antibody to the toxic conformation of tau, cis-tau. In animal studies, repeated concussions lead to the formation of cis-tau. This cis-tau is toxic to brain cells and is associated with abnormal behavior in the animals. Furthermore, even when the injuries are stopped, as the animals age this cis-tau spreads throughout their brain. The antibody developed by doctors Lu and Zhou prevents the spread of cis-tau throughout the brain, and this is associated with better outcomes, both on a cellular level and a functional level. Therefore, this represents a potential treatment for CTE, as far as the abnormal form of tau, cis-tau, is responsible for the symptoms of those diagnosed with it.

Exercise as Treatment

As has been noted throughout, the recommendations for recovery after a sport-related concussion were often to rest the body physically by avoiding exercise until full resolution of symptoms. Recent research has suggested that low intensity exercise is not harmful and may in fact be beneficial during recovery from concussion. Preliminary data suggest that those who engage in low risk, low level aerobic exercise that does not exacerbate their symptoms may suffer less symptoms and shorter recovery times than those who engage in complete rest. It is likely that continuation of this research will show that low-level exercise is in fact beneficial for those recovering from concussion.

Part of the reason for that may have to do with the disruption of blood flow to the brain and its regulatory mechanisms in the body. Preliminary research has shown the way blood flow to the brain is regulated is disrupted when people who are used to remove exercising regularly suddenly stop. This is true even in the absence of a concussion. This disruption of the mechanisms of the regulation of blood flow to the brain can lead to symptoms such as low energy, dizziness, headaches, and other problems often caused by and attributed to concussion. Therefore, it could be that some of the symptoms athletes experience after concussion may be due to the fact that they went from exercising regularly to suddenly stopping exercise, as opposed to the cellular changes caused by the concussion itself.

Causes of CTE

The initial hypotheses regarding the cause of CTE based on the initial cases reported suggested that sport-related concussions led to the changes on the cellular level. This hypothesis has been strengthened by the overall number of cases of CTE that have been diagnosed among those who experienced repetitive trauma to the brain, such as athletes in collision and contact sports, as well as military personnel who sustained injuries during battle. Furthermore, animal models have confirmed that repeated blows to the brain will result in the formation of the abnormal conformation of the protein tau that leads to hyperphosphorylation that is associated with CTE. It is difficult, however, to tell whether this abnormal protein results from concussions themselves or potentially even subconcussive blows, those blows to the head that do not result in the signs and symptoms necessary to diagnose a concussion. There have been athletes found to have hyperphosphorylated tau in their brains after death that had never been diagnosed with a concussion. It is, however, difficult to diagnose a concussion, particularly among athletes, as research has shown that many athletes are reluctant to report their injuries for fear of losing play time or for not recognizing their symptoms as being due to a concussion. Therefore, it remains unclear whether these abnormal protein deposits resulted from concussions that were unreported or from subconcussive blows.

It is also difficult to answer this question using animal models, as animals cannot report their symptoms. Therefore, the only way to know whether a blow to the head has resulted in a concussion or not is to check if they have physical, measurable signs of concussion. One can imagine that an animal may suffer symptoms such as headaches, dizziness, and nausea without any physical signs of concussion that are observable to a laboratory technician. Therefore, assuming that a blow is subconcussive when there are not physical signs of concussion could be erroneous.

Furthermore, in one of the largest studies of CTE to date, a Canadian pathologist named Shawna Noy, and her colleagues stained the brains of more than 100 people who showed up in the pathology lab for hyperphosphorylated tau. The study showed that a history of trauma to the head was a risk factor for the presence of hyperphosphorylated tau. But substance abuse, including alcohol abuse, was also a risk factor for the presence of hyperphosphorylated tau, even in the absence of head trauma. Furthermore, approximately 20 percent of people who had no history of substance abuse and no history of head trauma also stained positive for the presence of hyperphosphorylated tau. Therefore, there may be other risk factors besides sport-related concussion that can cause CTE that are discovered in the future.

In summary, there is a substantial amount of research in the area of sport-related concussion that is ongoing. In the future, we may be able to predict whether certain people are at risk for concussion or at risk for poor outcomes after sustaining repeated sport-related concussions. We may have better treatments for concussion itself and for the potential effects of repeated sport-related concussions, up to and including CTE. We may have better ways to make the diagnosis either through imaging or through markers found in the blood, urine, or saliva. It is worth noting, however, that the title of this chapter is, *The Future.* As such, all the information contained in this chapter should be considered preliminary, and while thought provoking, it is not yet clinically applicable or useful. Any information in this chapter that you think might be applicable to you or a loved one should be discussed with a physician skilled and experienced in the management of sport-related concussion.

SUGGESTED READINGS

Albalawi, T., J.W. Hamner, M. Lapointe, W. Meehan, and C.O. Tan. The relationship between cerebral vasoreactivity and post-concussive symptom severity. *J Neurotrauma,* 2017 [Epub ahead of print].

Anderson, R.E., et al. High serum S100B levels for trauma patients without head injuries. *Neurosurgery,* 2001, 48(6): 1255–1258; discussion 1258–1260.

Biberthaler, P., et al. Serum S-100B concentration provides additional information for the indication of computed tomography in patients after minor head injury: A prospective multicenter study. *Shock,* 2006, 25(5): 446–453.

Chen, J.K., et al. A validation of the post concussion symptom scale in the assessment of complex concussion using cognitive testing and functional MRI. *J Neurol Neurosurg Psychiatry,* 2007, 78(11): 1231–1238.

Collins, M.W., et al. Relationship between postconcussion headache and neuropsychological test performance in high school athletes. *Am J Sports Med,* 2003, 31(2): 168–173.

de Kruijk, J.R., et al. S-100B and neuron-specific enolase in serum of mild traumatic brain injury patients. A comparison with health controls. *Acta Neurol Scand,* 2001, 103(3): 175–179.

Grool, A.M., M. Aglipay, F. Momoli, W.P. Meehan III, S.B. Freedman, K.O. Yeates, J. Gravel, I. Gagnon, K. Boutis, W. Meeuwisse, N. Barrowman, M.H. Osmond, and R. Zemek, on behalf of the Pediatric Emergency Research Canada (PERC) Concussion Team. Association between early participation in physical activity following acute pediatric concussion and persistent post-concussive symptoms in children and adolescents. *J Am Med Assoc,* 2016, 316(23): 2504–2514.

Guskiewicz, K.M., et al. Measurement of head impacts in collegiate football players: Relationship between head impact biomechanics and acute clinical outcome after concussion. *Neurosurgery,* 2007, 61(6): 1244–1252; discussion 1252–1253.

Howell, D.R., R.C. Mannix, B. Quinn, J.A. Taylor, C.O. Tan, and W.P. Meehan III. Physical activity level and symptom duration are not associated after concussion. *Am J Sports Med,* 2016, 44(4): 1040–1046.

Iverson, G.L., et al. Relation between subjective fogginess and neuropsychological testing following concussion. *J Int Neuropsychol Soc*, 2004, 10(6): 904–906.

Jordan, B.D., et al. Apolipoprotein E epsilon4 associated with chronic traumatic brain injury in boxing. JAMA, 1997, 278(2): 136–140.

Khuman, J., Meehan, W.P. III., Zhu, X. et al. TNF-α and fas receptors mediate cognitive deficits independent of cell death after closed head injury in mice. In Second Joint Symposium of International and National Neurotrauma Societies, 2009.

Kondo, A., et al. Antibody against early driver of neurodegeneration cis P-tau blocks brain injury and tauopathy. *Nature*, 2015, 523(7561): 431–436.

Liberman, J.N., et al. Apolipoprotein E epsilon 4 and short-term recovery from predominantly mild brain injury. *Neurology*, 2002, 58(7): 1038–1044.

Linstedt, U., et al. Serum concentration of S-100 protein in assessment of cognitive dysfunction after general anesthesia in different types of surgery. *Acta Anaesthesiol Scand*, 2002, 46(4): 384–389.

Mannix, R.C., et al. Age-dependent effect of apolipoprotein E4 on functional outcome after controlled cortical impact in mice. *J Cereb Blood Flow Metab* 2011, 31(1): 351–61.

Mayeux, R., et al. Synergistic effects of traumatic head injury and apolipoprotein-epsilon 4 in patients with Alzheimer's disease. *Neurology*, 1995, 45(3 Pt 1): 555–557.

McCrory, P., et al. Consensus statement on concussion in sport: The Fifth International Conference on Concussion in Sport held in Berlin, October 2016. *Br J Sports Med*, 2017 [Epub ahead of print].

Meehan, W.P., III, A.M. Taylor, P. Berkner, N.J. Sandstrom, M. Peluso, M.M. Kurtz, A. Pascual-Leone, and R. Mannix. Division III collision sports are not associated with neurobehavioral quality-of-life. *J Neurotrauma*, 2016, 33(2): 254–259.

Mei, Z., J. Qiu, S. Alcon, J. Hashim, A. Rotenberg, Y. Sun, W.P. Meehan III, and R. Mannix. Memantine improves outcomes after repetitive traumatic brain injury. *Behav Brain Res* [Epub ahead of print].

Pelinka, L.E., et al. Circulating S100B is increased after bilateral femur fracture without brain injury in the rat. *Br J Anaesth*, 2003, 91(4): 595–597.

Teasdale, G.M., et al. Association of apolipoprotein E polymorphism with outcome after head injury. *Lancet*, 1997, 350(9084): 1069–1071.

17

In Their Own Words: Athletes from the Sports Concussion Clinic of Boston Children's Hospital

Since cofounding the Sports Concussion Clinic in the Division of Sports Medicine at Children's Hospital Boston, I have been privileged to care for some wonderful young athletes. Fortunately, most have recovered quickly, without complications. But others have suffered through long, frustrating recoveries. Some were plagued by repetitive head injuries, despite refraining from contact and collision sports. For some, their injuries changed their lives, their network of friends, and their academic performance. I can think of no better way to conclude this book than to have some of these exceptional athletes describe their own experiences with concussions and relay to the readers how their injuries affected their lives.

Furthermore, the occurrence of repeated sport-related concussions can affect more than just the athlete himself. It also affects teammates, coaches, friends, and in particular, parents. Often the decision to decide whether an athlete should return to sports after suffering multiple concussions is difficult both for the athlete as well as the athlete's parents who are always involved in that decision when it is a pediatric athlete. Therefore, in this new edition of this book, I am delighted to include the story of a mother, herself a physician, who had to make the difficult decision of whether to allow her son to continue to participate in sports after he suffered multiple sport-related concussions.

CHARLIE COOK

Pain, hopelessness, fear, anger. These were the only companions I had when I tried to sleep in my dark, quiet bedroom where the silence was deafening. They worked hard during that time trying to define me, and I was pretty sure that they were going to succeed in their quest. I was a freshman in high school when I got my last concussion, and I was just too tired or too scared or maybe even just too lazy to fight my way back to normalcy again.

I have played all sports since I was very young, and some of my concussions were caused by athletic injuries. Others were the results of unfortunate mishaps, but each set of headaches that were a result of my concussions were progressive and they were worst pain I had ever felt in my entire life. The pain was sharp, yet dull and constant, but intermittent. The headaches incapacitated me so much that all I was able to do was just lay in bed in a dark room for days. The pain from the headaches was so severe at times that even sleep was elusive and I would just lay there and worry about my future. The fear that my brain might never heal was more incapacitating than the headaches and then anger would envelop me. I was angry about the pain, angry that I missed so many high school experiences, angry that I had missed so many athletic opportunities and mostly angry that I was not going to cherish the memories that had not yet even happened.

I would like to say that I had a revelation one day and decided to battle my demons with courage and strength, but this is not my personality. My condition improved both spontaneously and also because of intensive medical care over time and I was able to concentrate, study, maintain my grades, and return to the athletic field and my social life. I have been reassured by my physicians that I am cleared to play sports and to participate in any event that I choose to do. I look back at that dark time and realize that instead of attacking my demons, I just chose to ignore them and pushed through the complications of my concussions on a minute-to-minute basis. I changed my way of learning using a verbal approach instead of a written approach and the hopelessness started to lessen. I began to exercise again and the comforting, sweet smell of sweat cut through my anger. I learned to cope with the pain of the headaches and although I was still afraid of my future, it was a little easier to at least think about it. I did battle, but my battle was not inspirational for anyone but me. I realize that I am not a hero and I also realize that other teenagers have had to overcome much worse medical issues than concussions. However, I also realize that my methods may not be pretty or dramatic, but I can and will overcome obstacles and ultimately succeed in life. It was a lesson hard learned, but one worth the journey.

I think concussions are extremely misunderstood injuries and are very difficult to treat. We have all seen the negative effects and long-term symptoms concussions can bring if an athlete chooses to continue playing without taking the time for allowing the concussions to heal, but no one has actually looked at the flip side of asking an athlete to stop playing their sport all together. As someone who has had several concussions over lifetime, I have experienced all the bad effects of being out of sports during recovery. It is good to rest and try to recover after sustaining a concussion to try to lessen the symptoms, but being out of sports has its downsides as well. My time away from sports was an extremely difficult time in my life. Sports had a huge role in my life growing up and having that taken away from me was unbearable. Watching my friends and teammates participate while I had to watch from the sidelines was very tough because I wanted to be out there so badly. I felt cheated and angry that they had the opportunity to continue playing, but that opportunity was completely taken away from me. I feel like I lost many friends during the time I was out of sports simply because I wasn't spending nearly as much time with those friends as I was when I was playing sports. Another disadvantage of not being able to play sports was that I gained a large amount of weight by not exercising as much. I would say that both of these downsides set me back socially and physically for many years. However, I am back playing lacrosse for the high school and basketball for fun, and this has allowed me to make up for lost time by slowly getting back into shape and reuniting with old friends. Playing sports again has also helped me dramatically with my future. If I wasn't playing lacrosse, I probably wouldn't have been going to a very good academic college next year. I will be attending Clark University after committing to play lacrosse next year and I know for sure that I would not have been accepted at such a great college if it wasn't playing lacrosse. I can't thank Dr. Meehan enough for helping me through all this. I have now been his patient for seven years, and he has taken the time to get to know me as a person, so he realized just how much I needed to play sports again because he treated me as a kid with other social and physical issues and not just a kid with multiple concussions.

Maureen Cook, Mother and Physician

As a physician and more importantly, as a mother of two boys who loved contact sports, I learned early in their lives to not overreact to any of their athletic injuries. However, I was very worried and will always be worried about my youngest son, Charlie, who has sustained six documented concussions. He was a big, strong, and athletic kid who really excelled at football and lacrosse. He received his first three concussions by jumping off a couch, colliding with a classmate while trying to save a basketball from going out of bounds, and getting kicked in the head during a pick up football game. These three concussions left him with really no symptoms and he returned to sports and his normal life pretty quickly. However, his fourth concussion occurred when he was in the eighth grade playing football for the Middle School football team. He then stopped playing all sports for one year. Despite that being a tough year, he remained a very outgoing, engaged, popular kid who maintained his friendships with the other athletes in his class because he was told that he could return to lacrosse and football after taking a break from these sports after a year. He then returned to freshman football, but almost immediately received a fifth concussion.

Charlie had been seeing Dr. Meehan for almost three and a half years at that time. Together, we decided that Charlie should not return to football or lacrosse ever again. It was then that he began to change his personality.

However, he then had improvement in his concussion symptoms by the spring of his freshman year. He was not clinically depressed at that time, but he became much more quiet and reserved and he also began to lose contact with his friends because they continued playing sports, but Charlie was unable to do this. Because he became even more withdrawn and because he missed participating in sports so much, Charlie then joined the track team in the spring of his freshman year. He then sustained his sixth concussion when he was hit with a shot put ball during an indoor practice. He then had even worse post-concussion symptoms, but by the fall of his sophomore year, the symptoms again improved. At that time, he tried to participate in Cross Country, but because he is big and strong but also very slow, he was basically "cut" from the team. He continued to work hard academically, but he gained weight due to the lack of exercise with sports and he seemed to withdraw even further. Although he wasn't using drugs or alcohol, he just "went through the motions" and seemed to lack emotion. Finally, by the spring of his sophomore year, it had been three years since Charlie had participated in either lacrosse or football and he desperately wanted to return playing either or both of them. After working with Dr. Meehan, Charlie was advised to avoid football, but he was allowed to return to lacrosse as a goalie, which had been his position when he was younger.

Since returning to lacrosse, Charlie has completely reverted to his old self. He has lost some weight, made new friends, rekindled old friendships, is happy, active, and outgoing. He is now a senior in high school and has also done well in lacrosse. He has been recruited by several colleges and is currently the captain of the high school team. He committed to playing lacrosse at Clark University in Worcester, MA, and he and I both agree that he would not have been accepted to Clark without the help of lacrosse.

Charlie is very happy with his decision because lacrosse definitely helped him with the acceptance process at Clark. As a mother, I still wonder what would have happened to him had he not returned to lacrosse. I still wonder if he would have become clinically depressed, abused drugs and alcohol, or dropped out of high school. I know that this may sound dramatic, but as a mother, I was just so worried because he became such a different person when he was told that he could never return to the sports he loved. As a mother, my decision to allow Charlie to play lacrosse again was one of the best "Mom" decisions I have ever made.

Amanda Giambanco

My name is Amanda Giambanco, I am 17 years old, and I am a senior at Mansfield High School. I have been playing softball since I was in first grade. Over the years of playing, I have played many positions and had fun until I got into high school. When I entered high school, I really needed to focus one position, so I picked right field. I was on the JV team freshman year, and sophomore, junior, and senior year I was on varsity. When I moved up to varsity my sophomore year, I knew I was going to have to try a little harder than I had been. Even though I did not play in the field my first year, I still pinch ran for the pitcher every time she got on base. At the time there was a senior who was playing right field, so I knew that I would not play over her. With that mind-set I went to every practice and game and tried my hardest, put in the most effort that I could to try to show the coach I was good enough. My junior year, the senior that played right field had graduated high school, so there was a position open. Due to the fact that I always came to the games and practices with a good attitude and tried my hardest, my coach gave me the starting position in right field. I played every game my junior year, and we also made it to tournament that year. We moved on to the second to last round and ended up losing to Silver Lake. Although it was sad we lost, I knew I had another year to play and another chance to win the tournament.

Going into my senior year, after the first five games, our record was 4–1, so we had won four games and lost one. Our next game was on a Saturday and we were playing Needham. We got on the bus really early to get to the game. As soon as we got to the game, it started to rain and it got really cold, but we still played. I started in right field and started 7th in the batting order. We were in the 5th inning and we were up by a lot. The girl who was up before me hit a single so she had gotten on base. When I got up I ended up getting on base due to the pitcher hitting me with the pitch. The girl behind me hit a double, which put me on third. The next batter was up and there were two out. The girl hit the ball to the right side of the field, so I took off running home. As I got to home plate, I was running as fast as I can, slipped on the plate with my metal cleats, and went head first into the ground. Although the helmet on my head was there, it did not stop my brain from moving. The rest of the game I sat on the bench having a headache instantly. As I went home that day, my headache did not go away. After three days, my headache did not go away so I went to the doctors. At the pediatrician, he told me that I had a concussion. At this point I was upset because I did not want to sit out of softball my senior year. Because this was my third concussion, my doctor sent me to Dr. Meehan at Children's Hospital in Boston. The next day we went to see him, and he told me rest for a few days and gradually return to school and exercise. After a few weeks I went back to Dr. Meehan to check in with him on how I was doing. Although I didn't have a headache that day, within the past weeks I was still getting headaches at night, and I had to be honest and tell him. As soon as I told him that I knew it was going to be bad news. At this time I had missed the softball season and we had five games left. As I was sitting there, he told me I still could not play yet, because of my headaches. When he told me this, it was very upsetting because I wanted to play. I went easy with activity that week and then went back to Dr. Meehan the following Thursday. When I met with him this time, I had no headaches. I went into a room by myself to take the ImPACT test, and I passed. I was so excited when

I heard him say that I could play again. I finished the season with the team and we made tournament again.

Laura Schissler

For as long as I can remember, sports were a large part of how I defined myself with many of my childhood memories consisting of playing fields and practices. By the time I entered sixth grade, my main sports were lacrosse, soccer, and hockey, and it was clear I tied my sense-of-identity to athletics. Playing on boys' teams as I grew up further augmented my level of confidence while making me feel powerful and fearless even as a five-foot, shrimp of a girl.

I sustained my first concussion when I was 12 years old while playing ice hockey. During an unusually rough game, I was hit in the head multiple times until the point that I felt sick. In this sense, my injury strayed from what people typically believe has to occur during a head injury: blacking out. Consequently, I did not leave the game nor did my coach remove me as neither of us knew at the time what I was experiencing was a brain injury. In the locker room following the game, my mom was merely told "Laura does not feel well," leaving it up to her to decide what to do. Fortunately we took a trip to Boston Children's Hospital where I began treatment under the care of Dr. Meehan. I experienced many common symptoms of concussions: confusion, dizziness, sensitivity to light and sound, and nausea. There were many setbacks that had the potentially to deter my hope for feeling "normal" again; however, Dr. Meehan's reassurance and encouragement that I would once again reach my baseline fueled my determination. What starkly separates concussions from other types of injuries is the invisibility factor; although I looked okay to most, on the inside I felt terrible. That made it especially challenging to explain to coaches, teachers, and friends what exactly is wrong and why I could not participate in certain activities.

During my next hockey season I suffered another brain injury occurring during practice after I hit the back of my head on the goal post during a drill. I did not experience severe symptoms immediately following the incident, but rather after a delayed period of time. This made it especially confusing; when the throbbing headache and fatigue began I could not recall how or when I could have suffered a brain injury. Because the injury was not remarkable, when I explained how I was feeling to others, no one entertained the idea of another concussion; I was told I probably had a virus. As a result, my treatment was delayed, making the symptoms of the second concussion far more acute and persistent, lasting for over several months. The experience was especially frustrating, as I had to restrain from physical activity and mentally could not focus or concentrate. Consequently, I was out of school for one-third of the year and required tutoring at home. I slept for a majority of the day and missed out on many fun, social activities. When I did attend school, I would find myself needing breaks and overwhelmed with my inability to focus. Even months later, the aftereffects of the injury were apparent: slower reflexes, tentative movements, concentration issues, and depression. Eventually I recovered after many visits to Dr. Meehan, a specialized training program, and months of rest. Unbelievably, I experienced another concussion the following year during my soccer season from a kick to the temple inside the goal box. We sought treatment right away, and I again followed the protocol. At this point after three concussions, I was discouraged and dubious if I would ever return to sports. Dr. Meehan guided me through my options regarding my future in athletics, always honest about my increased risks balanced with encouragement that I could still participate in sports.

With the recommendations from Dr. Meehan taken into consideration, I slowly eased into athletics during high school beginning with becoming a team manager and decided to dedicate myself to only one contact sport. I also explored other options that posed less risk of a head injury during other seasons. As a manager, I built relationships with my teammates and coaches yet it was difficult still feeling handicapped by my medical history.

Although I was extremely lucky to recover, the brain injuries I sustained were life-altering as student and athlete and taught me a lot about myself. I found that, just like the challenges that test your strength in action on a field, adversity and recovery test your mental and physical perseverance as well. As a kid who defined myself through the sports I played, suddenly finding myself on the sidelines pushed me to discover other passions and mediums to express who I am.

ALYSSA PAUL

I have hit my head a time or two. Through playing soccer, basketball, and softball for 16 years, I have seen several athletes get a concussion or need to go to the hospital after a hard hit. I never thought that a quick shoulder to the chin at basketball practice would give me a concussion.

When I got my concussion, I was taking a charge when my teammate's shoulder and my chin collided, quite hard I might add. As soon as it happened, I knew something was off. Besides the blaring headache, I felt like I was in a blur and couldn't focus. As soon as my team broke the huddle and we were leaving the gym, I became extremely emotional for no apparent reason. I approached my coach and told her, "I think I have a concussion." We both were unsure that I had suffered as severe an injury as I suspected, in light of the fact that both of us had never seen a concussion resulting from what we thought was a lower-level impact compared to what we had both witnessed in the past. Typically, concussed athletes usually can't remember their name, the date, or even count to ten. My symptoms were much different, but when I got back to my apartment I couldn't even open my eyes.

My school is fortunate enough to have a very good athletic training staff, who came in the next morning to evaluate me. Immediately, my trainer said that I was unlike myself; my eyes were barely open, and I had poor balance. The trainer had a high degree of suspicion that I had suffered a concussion and needed to go into "shut down mode." The athletic trainers were following their long-established concussion protocol that requires athletes to completely refrain from all activity for the first seven days of concussion recovery. The first two to four days are shut down; no phone, low light, and no school work. Depending on how I felt after those initial days, I could be introduced to more light and activities, eventually leading to increased school work and exercise. However, my case was a little different. My initial headache lasted much longer than the required "shut down" period of time, and the trainers were not comfortable allowing me to do more, worrying about further injury.

With a rigorous academic calendar as an engineering student and the start of the semester approaching, I was fortunate to have the opportunity to have an appointment with Dr. Michael O'Brien at the Micheli Center for Sports Injury Prevention. After several cognitive tests, Dr. O'Brien sat with me for an hour and explained how he wanted to treat this concussion. He explained to me that recent studies are leaning toward recovering with more activity versus the "shut down" mode theory. Dr. O'Brien explained that an athlete at my level begins to feel tired, grouchy, and get a headache when we take an extended period of time off from exercise. I left the office with a specific timeline of how to gradually get back into school and noncontact basketball through maintaining a balance between no activity and normal activity levels. Following his plan, I found that I could do more and more exercise and classwork every day. Within the next two weeks, I saw a *huge* improvement in my concussion symptoms. At first, it was hard to get myself out the door or to sit in class, but eventually it became easier and easier. Becoming active while I had a concussion versus sitting in my room (like I had been) made the difference for me.

The detailed plan that Dr. O'Brien gave me, initially allowed me to walk a short distance as my exercise, do only 10 minutes of homework at a time, and I had to keep sunglasses on and earplugs in. The doctor made it clear that I keep my heartrate below the point where I was breathing through my mouth. After I could complete that without an increasing headache, I was allowed to gradually step up to jogging and 20- to 30-minute periods of homework. As my headache became less and less frequent, I progressed to light weightlifting, sprinting, and full days of classes. The final step was to try a non-contact practice to see how my body responded. After making it through all the steps Dr. O'Brien had given me, I was finally cleared to fully participate in both school and basketball.

My professors, coaches, and trainers understood that I would have to ease into work/practice in a much different way than the accepted norm for our training staff. My school also has a great resource in the Office of Disability Services, which allowed me to have extra time on exams and access to professor notes. My recovery process would not have been possible without their cooperation.

The doctor made it clear to me that little to no exercise for an athlete can be detrimental, especially in a concussed athlete. I was so glad to be able to participate in more activity; my coaches, my team, and my parents were proud of me when I finally worked up to being able to run! This method of recovery helped me get back into my classes and schoolwork, basketball, and feel like myself again!

SUGGESTED READINGS

Bailes, J. *Sports-Related Concussion*. St. Louis, MO: Quality Medical Publishing, 1999.

Mason, M. *Head Cases: Stories of Brain Injury and Its Aftermath*. New York: Farrar, Straus and Giroux, 2008.

Nowinski, C. *Head Games: Football's Concussion Crisis*. East Bridgewater, MA: The Drummond Publishing Group, 2007.

18

DEFINITIONS AND TEAM MEMBERS: UNDERSTANDING WHO WILL HELP CARE FOR THE ATHLETE WITH A SPORT-RELATED CONCUSSION

It will be helpful for the reader to understand certain terms that are used frequently in sports, sports medicine, and in the management of sport-related concussions. Similarly, the various medical personnel involved in assessing and managing sport-related concussions will be unfamiliar to those outside the medical field and to those who are not well acquainted with sports. Therefore, each is described below.

PERSONNEL

Clinician

Clinician is a general term for a medical professional who assesses and treats patients with an illness or injury. Doctors, nurses, psychologists, neuropsychologists, nurse practitioners, athletic trainers, physician assistants, and many others are all included under the term "clinician."

Athletic Trainer

A certified athletic trainer (ATC) is a medically trained professional who specializes in the assessment and treatment sport-related injuries. Oftentimes, each team will have its own athletic trainer or even several athletic trainers, who oversee the health care of the athletes. When an athlete is injured, it is the athletic trainer who is usually the first medical professional to respond. The athletic trainer will have the athlete explain how the injury occurred. He or she will examine the athlete and decide whether further management is needed. Often, the athletic trainer alone will treat the injury. Athletic trainers have expertise in certain types of treatment, as well as in taping and bracing techniques, which can prevent injury or allow an athlete with a mild injury to continue to participate in sports. Athletic trainers are an essential part of the sports medicine team. Since their specialty is sport-related injuries, athletic trainers, in general, will know a great deal about sport-related concussion. They will often know as much, if not more, about sport-related concussions than other medical specialists who do not have an interest in sports medicine or concussive brain injury.

Sports Medicine Doctor

A sports medicine doctor has completed extra medical training focused on the illnesses and injuries of athletes, and how athletes are affected by illness and injury. Sports medicine doctors specialize in the assessment, management, and treatment of sport-related injuries. There are two types of sports medicine doctors: sports medicine physicians and sports medicine surgeons. Sports medicine surgeons are doctors who initially trained in orthopedic surgery, and then went on to do specialty training in sport-related surgery. They can perform many surgeries arthroscopically. That means, instead of cutting a joint open in order to reconstruct a ligament, repair an injured meniscus, or tend to other injured structures, they can make small incisions through which they insert a camera and other small tools needed for repairing or reconstructing injured structures. Such small incisions allow for quicker recovery times. Often, athletes who undergo arthroscopic surgery are able to return to sports sooner than those who undergo open surgeries. In addition to performing surgery, sports medicine surgeons are able to assess and treat many sport-related injuries, mostly involving the bones, muscles, tendons, and ligaments of athletes. Should an athlete sustain an injury which requires surgery, it is best performed by a sports medicine surgeon. I should point out, that not all surgeries can be performed arthroscopically. However, a surgeon trained in sports medicine will know which procedure is best for the athlete, allowing the athlete to safely return to play at his or her prior level of performance, in the shortest possible amount of time.

Sports medicine physicians are doctors who initially trained in a medical field such as internal medicine, pediatrics, family practice, or emergency medicine. After their initial training, they went on to do more specialized training in the assessment and management of sport-related injuries. While they will also treat injuries related to bone, muscle, tendons, and ligaments, they will also treat many other illnesses suffered by athletes. As sport-related concussion is a common injury in athletes, these physicians will be educated and knowledgeable about the assessment and management of sport-related concussions.

Team Physician

The team physician is a doctor who is dedicated to work with a specific athletic team. For professional, college, and many other teams with significant resources, this doctor will almost always be one who is trained in sports medicine. However, for those teams without such resources, this may be a physician or an orthopedic surgeon who has an interest in sports and takes care of the athletes without having any specific training in sports medicine. Frequently, the team physician manages not only the athletic injuries of the team, but also other common ailments and illnesses that arise throughout the year, such as influenza outbreaks and chronic conditions of the athletes such as asthma.

Neuropsychologist

A neuropsychologist is a scientist and clinician who specializes in the assessment of brain function. Neuropsychologists have earned either a doctor of psychology degree (PsyD) or a doctor of philosophy degree (PhD). When a neuropsychologist sees a patient, he or she will ask the patient to perform certain tasks which help the neuropsychologist measure elements of brain function. In the setting of sport-related concussion, neuropsychologists are used for several purposes. Sometimes, they will administer neuropsychological tests prior to the start of the sports season in order to obtain what is known as a "baseline" measurement of brain function. These are measurements of brain function that are taken before an athlete has sustained a concussion. They can be used to assess changes in brain function after a concussive injury occurs. In addition, neuropsychologists are called upon to measure brain function after injury. This may either be to help determine whether an athlete has sustained a sport-related concussion or whether an athlete has recovered from a known sport-related concussion. For those athletes who are unfortunate enough to have a slow recovery from their sport-related concussions, the neuropsychologist will often use measurements of brain function to help determine the athlete's abilities. For student-athletes, neuropsychologists will often devise an academic plan that helps the athlete learn despite the limitations of brain function resulting from the injury. Neuropsychologists will provide treatments and strategies to help athletes with their recoveries.

Nurse Practitioner

A nurse practitioner (NP) is a nurse who has gone on to do extra medical training. Nurse practitioners are able to evaluate patients, order tests, make diagnoses, and prescribe treatments for those diagnoses, including medications. They act, in many ways, like physicians. But they have not undergone the same training as a doctor and do not have an MD degree.

Physician Assistant

A physician assistant (PA or PA-C for physician assistant, certified) is similar to a nurse practitioner. A physician assistant has completed medical training that allows him or her to evaluate patients, order tests, make diagnoses, and prescribe treatments for those diagnoses, including medications. They too act in many ways like a physician, but have not undergone the same training as doctors and do not have an MD degree.

Primary Care Physician

Primary care physicians are the doctors that most readers will be familiar with. These are physicians who have trained in internal medicine, pediatrics or family practice. Unlike the sports medicine physicians, these doctors have not completed extra medical training in the assessment and management of sport-related injuries. However, many will take an active interest in managing athletes. Some of these physicians will be up to date on the current medical literature regarding sport-related concussion. Some will have all the available resources to properly treat these athletes. It is these physicians who provide care to most athletes who sustain a sport-related concussion. If sport-related concussion is not an injury that a certain primary care physician is confident managing, or if a particular athlete or injury is medically complicated, the primary care physician may consult with other doctors who have more specialized training in the assessment and management of sport-related concussions or concussive brain injuries in general.

Neurosurgeon

A neurosurgeon is a surgeon who specializes in performing operations on the skull, brain, spine, and spinal cord. Although concussion is not an injury that requires surgery, many neurosurgeons will be familiar with the assessment and management of concussions. Many will manage these athletes. Those who do not will certainly be familiar with other clinicians in their area who manage sport-related concussions.

Neurologist

Neurologists are doctors who specialize in the diseases and illnesses that affect the nerves of the body and brain. Although concussive brain injury is not typically a part of neurology training, some will have taken an active interest in this area, and can assess and manage a sport-related concussion. More often, these highly skilled physicians will be called upon to assist in the management of post-concussive headaches, headaches that occur after a concussion. At Children's Hospital Boston, we are fortunate to have several neurologists with an interest in concussive brain injury.

Psychologist/Sports Psychologist

Psychologists are clinicians who specialize in treating emotional disturbances and behavioral problems. They use counseling as the main therapy.

They are often able to provide certain strategies which help people manage their emotional and behavioral problems. A sports psychologist is a psychologist who has taken specialized training and has an active interest in those psychological problems that affect athletes and athletic performance. In the setting of sport-related concussion, sports psychologists are often used to help athletes cope with their injuries and the limitations on their life that result from concussive brain injury.

Psychiatrist

A psychiatrist is a physician who specializes in the assessment and management of mental illness. In the setting of sport-related concussions, a psychiatrist may be consulted to help manage the depression experienced by some athletes who suffer a prolonged recovery after sustaining a sport-related concussion. These cases are rare. For most athletes recovering from a sport-related concussion, psychiatric medications will not be indicated.

School Nurse

The school nurse is often one of the first clinicians to assess an athlete who has sustained a sport-related concussion. Some schools are not fortunate enough to have an athletic trainer. Other times, the athletic trainer may be on the road with a team that has an away game. Therefore, athletes injured during a home game will be taken to the school nurse. As sport-related concussions draw more and more attention both in the medical literature and in the popular media, school nurses are being called upon more frequently help coordinate the assessment and management of sport-related concussions.

TERMS

Cognitive Function

"Cognitive" is a medical term used to describe certain functions of the brain. Cognitive function refers to those functions of the brain which involve thinking, concentrating, learning, and reasoning. Throughout much of the medical literature, the terms "cognitive," neurocognitive," and "neuropsychological" are often used interchangeably. While there are, in fact, subtle differences in their meaning, such details are not necessary for understanding this book nor relevant for most readers of this book. The terms may be considered similar in meaning for the sake of this text. Often, the term "brain function" will be used as a generic term to describe overall cognitive function.

Tasks that require cognitive effort include: reading, studying, videogame playing, working online, text messaging, playing games such as chess or Scrabble, and other similar activities.

Signs

When practicing medicine, we often refer to the *signs* and *symptoms* of an illness or injury. The *signs* of an illness or injury are those characteristics that can be observed by people other than the patient. For example, a rash would be a *sign* of illness. Swelling would be a *sign* of injury.

Symptoms

Symptoms, however, are those characteristics of an injury or illness that are experienced by the patients themselves. Nausea, for example, would be a *symptom* of an illness. Pain would be a *symptom* of an injury.

Amnesia

"Amnesia" is a medical term referring to a loss of memory, often caused by a traumatic injury to the brain.

Cervical Spine

Medically, the backbone is known as the spine. As opposed to being one long bone, the spine consists of multiple smaller bones stacked upon one another. The seven smaller bones of the spine that are located within the neck are known together as the cervical spine. The spine is important because it houses and protects the spinal cord, a set of nerves descending from the brain that control much of our bodily movements. Damage to the cervical spine can also result in damage to the spinal cord. This can lead to devastating consequences, including death and paralysis.

Sports Categories

Sports can be broken down into various categories. People often refer to "contact" sports. However, the meaning of this term is often unclear. Some will refer to both basketball and ice hockey as contact sports. However, it will be clear to most readers that the frequency of contact, the force of contact, and the intensity of contact that occurs during basketball is quite different than that which occurs during ice hockey. Therefore in this book, we will divide sports into three main categories:

1. Noncontact sports
2. Contact sports
3. Collision sports

Noncontact Sports

Noncontact sports are those in which contact with another player is neither an intentional nor an expected part of the game. Some common noncontact sports include tennis, cross-country running, track and field, and swimming.

Contact Sports

The term "contact sports" refers to those sports in which contact with another player is an expected part of the game. However, intentional blows to the body are not routinely delivered. Common contact sports are soccer, basketball, and baseball.

Collision Sports

Collision sports are those in which intentional body-to-body blows are part of the game. Common collision sports include American football, ice hockey, rugby, and lacrosse.

Combat Sports

Combat sports are a subset of collision sports. Most combat sports are one-on-one contests in which two combatants are engaged in a fight, albeit with a specific set of rules and regulations that are followed and monitored by a referee. Common combat sports are boxing, wrestling, karate, mixed martial arts, and other similar activities.

Trauma

"Trauma" refers to a wound or injury caused by a blow, collision, or force. Common examples of traumatic injuries are fractures, gunshot wounds, lacerations, bruises, and concussions.

Concussive Brain Injury

Concussive brain injury is another term for concussion. Concussive brain injury refers to an injury to the brain that, as we shall see, results from a rapid spinning or rotational acceleration of the brain.

Traumatic Brain Injury

The term "traumatic brain injury" refers to an injury to the brain that results from trauma, as defined above. There are other ways that the brain can be injured. For example, if somebody has a clot in one of their arteries such that blood cannot flow to the brain, the brain will sustain an injury from this lack of blood flow. Such an injury is more commonly referred to as a "stroke." This type of injury, however, is not due to trauma. When we discuss concussion, we are referring to a specific type of traumatic brain injury.

Mild Traumatic Brain Injury (mTBI)

Often the terms "concussion" and "mild traumatic brain injury" are used interchangeably. However, as many patients will attest, concussions are often far from "mild." Furthermore, while the terms concussion and concussive brain injury describe how the injury occurred, (that it resulted from a rapid spinning or rotational acceleration). The term mild traumatic brain injury does not specify the way in which the injury occurred. The term mild does not describe how significant the patient's symptoms are or how long it takes the patient to recover.

In fact, the term "mild" is solely determined by how the patient appears to the doctor at the time of injury. It is based on an evaluation of head trauma known as the Glasgow Coma Scale, commonly referred to as "GCS." The Glasgow Coma Scale is used by emergency medicine providers to communicate the level of consciousness of a patient who has sustained a trauma. The patient is given a number of points based on his or her response to various stimuli. Table 18.1 shows a version of the Glasgow Coma Scale, using common terminology.

Table 18.1
A Modified Version of the Glasgow Coma Scale

	Glasgow Coma Scale	
Motor response	The patient obeys commands	6
	The patient responds to a painful stimulus by moving toward the site of the stimulus	5
	The patient moves away from the a painful stimulus	4
	The patient flexes his or her joints in response to a painful stimulus	3
	The patients extends his or her joints in response to a painful stimulus	2
	The patient has no response to a painful stimulus	1

	Glasgow Coma Scale	
Verbal response	The patient is able to respond appropriately to questions regarding who he or she is and where he or she is	5
	The patient responds to questions, but is confused	4
	The patient responds to questioning using inappropriate words. There is no conversation	3
	The patient makes incomprehensible sounds, but no actual words	2
	No response to questioning	1
Eye opening	The patient spontaneously opens his or her eyes	4
	The patient opens his or her eyes to speech	3
	The patients opens his or her eyes to painful stimulus	2
	The patients does not open his or her eyes, despite painful stimulus	1
Total possible score		15

Patients are categorized mild if, when they arrive for medical care, they have a total score of 14 to 15 on the Glasgow Coma Scale. An uninjured person would typically have a score of 15.

While highly useful in the setting of emergency response to trauma, the Glasgow Coma Scale should not be used to assess the significance of a concussion. It does not predict how long it will take an athlete to recover from a concussion. Many patients who are diagnosed with "mild" traumatic brain injury, have diminished brain function, headaches, and other symptoms that last weeks or even months. Alternatively, some patients diagnosed with "moderate" traumatic brain injury will recover completely within days to weeks. Therefore, the term "mild traumatic brain injury" should not be used interchangeably with "concussion." Readers should understand that most concussions will recover rapidly, within hours or days. Other concussions, however, will result in symptoms that last months. At present, it is not possible to accurately predict which injuries will resolve rapidly, and which will result in more prolonged recovery.

Now that we have established the role of various medical personnel and described some of the terms commonly used during the assessment and treatment of sport-related concussions, we can talk in depth about sport-related concussions.

Suggested Readings

Bailes, J. *Sports-Related Concussion.* St. Louis, MO: Quality Medical Publishing, 1999.

Echemendia, R.J. *Sports Neuropsychology: Assessment and Management of Traumatic Brain Injury.* New York: The Guilford Press, 2006.

Lee, L.K. Consequences of trhe sequelae of pediatric mild traumatic brain injury. *Pediatric Emergency Care,* 2007, 23(8): 580–586.

Lovell, M.R., R.J. Echemendia, J.T. Barth, and M.W. Collins. *Traumatic Brain Injury in Sports: An International Neuropsychological Perspective.* Lisse, The Netherlands: Swets and Zeitlinger, 2004.

McCrea, M. *Mild Traumatic Brain Injury and Postconcussion Syndrome: The New Evidence Base for Diagnosis and Treatment.* New York: Oxford University Press, 2008.

Nowinski, C. *Head Games: Football's Concussion Crisis.* East Bridgewater, MA: The Drummond Publishing Group, 2007.

Appendix

BOSTON COLLEGE SPORTS MEDICINE[1] GUIDELINES FOR CARE OF THE CONCUSSED STUDENT-ATHLETE

This document is for use by Boston College Sports Medicine Clinicians when treating Student-Athletes (S-As) who have suffered a concussion or are suspected of having suffered a concussion. The term "mild traumatic brain injury" (mTBI) is not interchangeable with the term "concussion" and will not be used in this document.

POLICY GUIDELINES

Boston College maintains concussion care guidelines based on the most current research and consensus statements from noted experts around the world. This policy is reviewed yearly to ensure that we are following the most current standard of care and that the policy reflects new requirements dictated by both the National Collegiate Athletic Association (NCAA) and the City of Boston's Ordinance for College Athlete Head Injury Game Day Safety Protocol. There is no wording within the NCAA or Boston legislation that allows for "interpretation" by the clinician in regards to *initial care* of the S-A with a suspected head injury; this policy must be followed to ensure the safety of the S-A and to ensure that Boston College is compliant with NCAA and Boston regulations.

A concussion is considered a complex pathophysiological process affecting the brain, induced by traumatic biomechanical forces. This can be caused by a direct blow or impulsive forces transmitted to the head and typically results in a rapid onset of neurological impairments and clinical symptoms. A concussion is a functional injury, not a structural injury and may or may not include loss of consciousness (LOC). A concussion is not identifiable on standard imaging (CT, MRI).

---

[1]Used by permission.

At no time will any Sports Medicine clinician assign a "grade" to the concussive injury suffered by a S-A. Although there are a multitude of grading scales that have been created to assist in the diagnosis and management of concussion, these will not be employed by Boston College. Attempting to "slot" an S-As injury into one of these scales for the purpose of creating a care plan and a projected timeline places unnecessary restrictions and expectations on the clinician and is not the standard of care.

All NCAA varsity contact/collision sports sponsored by Boston College shall have medically trained personnel present at competitions (on site at campus or venue) and shall have medically trained personnel available for immediate consultation during any practice. These medically trained personnel shall be licensed and/or certified in the diagnosis, treatment and initial management of acute concussion. NCAA contact/collision sports sponsored by Boston College include M&W Basketball, Field Hockey, Football, M&W Ice Hockey, W. Lacrosse, M&W Skiing, and M&W Soccer.

Per requirements, any athlete who is deemed to have suffered a concussion, or is suspected of suffering a concussion after experiencing trauma shall be removed from all physical activity for the remainder of that calendar day. Boston College requires evaluation of the athlete, as soon as possible, by a Sports Medicine Clinician. If it is determined that the athlete has suffered a concussion, that athlete will be held from further activity and will be guided and monitored through the protocols outlined in this document. Return to play clearance will be determined by a team physician or appropriately trained and licensed health care clinician and will be documented in writing and provided to the Assistant Athletic Director for Sports Medicine.

The City of Boston Ordinance requires that, specifically for the sports of Football, Ice Hockey and Men's Lacrosse, a "Neurotrauma Consultant" be in attendance at any competition held within the City of Boston. By Ordinance definition, the Neurotrauma Consultant can be a neurologist or a "primary care CAQ sports medicine certified physician that has documented competence and experience in the treatment of acute head injuries." This physician shall have full access to benches and playing surface. Further, this physician will evaluate any suspected head, neck, or spine injury suffered by either a home or visiting athlete and will work with the medical staffs present to make recommendations for further care. If visiting teams have medical staff in attendance, they will make the final decision regarding the diagnosis and their athletes playing status.

Pre-Season Education

S-As in each sport will be presented with NCAA concussion fact sheets and educational material on concussions via "Jump Forward" from the compliance office and from pre-season compliance meetings *prior* to practice or competition. S-As will review the material with the understanding that they accept responsibility for reporting all of their injuries and illnesses to the medical staff, including signs and symptoms of concussions. Each S-A will initial and sign an acknowledgement of receipt, reading and understanding of concussion education.

Coaches, Sport Administrators, and the Athletics Director will be educated about concussions and the Concussion Safety Protocol as follows: Concussion education will be provided to coaches, Sport Oversight Administrators and the Athletics Director at the beginning of the academic year during an appropriate staff or compliance meeting. Coaches should understand their responsibility for helping to identify S-As exhibiting potential signs, symptoms or behaviors consistent with a concussion and getting them evaluated by the Athletic Trainer and/or Team Physician. Coaches will also be educated about strategies that reduce a S-A's exposure to head trauma. Coaches, Sports Administrators, and the Athletics Director will sign an acknowledgement of receipt, reading and understanding of concussion education.

Team Physicians and Athletic Trainers will also be provided concussion education material annually and will sign acknowledgement of receipt, reading and understanding of such material.

INITIAL AND BASELINE ASSESSMENT

All incoming freshmen and all new S-As will undergo a Sport Pre-Participation Physical through University Health Services. During this physical, the examining physician shall review the S-A's prior medical history including any history of brain injury or concussion as well as any current symptoms. Those S-As reporting prior head injury will be asked to provide a thorough history of their previous concussive incidents including dates incurred, length of symptoms, and time missed from athletics and academics. Each S-A will be administered a baseline Standard Assessment of Concussion. A balance screening shall also be administered by the examining physician or athletic training staff. Those S-As who are participating in contact and collision sports will also undergo computerized neurocognitive testing prior to participation. The Boston College sports that are classified as contact and collision are listed below. The results of these tests will be recorded in the S-A's medical chart. The examining physician will make a determination for clearance to participate or for the need of any type of specialized follow-up consultation related to pre-existing conditions and/or prior history of head injury.

The sports which will be required to undergo computerized neurocognitive baseline testing include:

Baseball	Field Hockey	W Lacrosse	M & W Skiing
M & W Basketball	Football	Pole Vaulting	Softball
Diving	M & W Ice Hockey	M & W Soccer	

Any athlete that has suffered a documented concussion and that has experienced a complicated, non-linear, or lengthy return to play progression, or has suffered multiple concussions while at Boston College shall undergo new baseline testing after six months (or longer) from the date of clearance.

EVALUATION/DIAGNOSIS

Signs and Symptoms of Concussion

Below is a list of signs and symptoms that may be used by the clinician to assist in the initial evaluation of the head injured S-A. This list is extensive but not all-inclusive and should serve only to provide "triggers" that may be used for identifying the S-A with a concussion. A similar, but more specific list will be utilized for follow-up with the concussed S-A. Understand that symptoms may vary over time and serial monitoring will occur regularly to further assess neurocognitive status. Re-evaluation is recommended daily in the initial post injury phase due to the variable sequelae that may ensue.

Physical	Cognitive	Emotional	Sleep
Headache	Difficulty remembering	Behavioral changes	Sleep more than usual
Fatigue	Difficulty concentrating	Irritability	Sleep less than usual
Dizziness	Feeling slowed down	Sadness	Drowsiness
Photophobia	Feeling in a fog	Feeling emotional	Trouble falling asleep
Sensitivity to noise	Slowed reaction times	Nervousness	
Nausea	Altered attention	Anxiety	
Balance problems	Amnesia		
LOC			
Vision difficulty			

Acute/Emergency Evaluation and Care (Sideline/ Bench—Immediately Post Injury)

At any time that a concussion is suspected, the S-A shall be removed from further participation and undergo an initial concussion evaluation.

If the S-A is conscious and alert and without evidence of other limiting injuries (i.e. c-spine injury), they will be removed to the sideline/bench/athletic training room for evaluation. At that time the clinician will, at a minimum, perform the following exam:

- The injury history, date/time, and history of previous concussion will be determined and recorded including any loss of consciousness
- An initial injury verbal symptom checklist will be utilized to record any symptoms reported by the S-A.
- A basic neurologic exam will take place assessing cranial nerves
- The SAC will be administered
- Upper and lower extremity coordination will be assessed.
- Pupils shall be examined for size, shape and reaction to light.

If the athlete is symptomatic and the clinician determines that the athlete is concussed, serial monitoring will occur at regular intervals (approx. every 10 minutes) until symptoms stabilize or improve. Serial monitoring will be recorded and should include time of day and any change in symptoms or status of athlete. Depending on sport, timing, and location, the helmet may be taken away from the injured player. Once symptoms stabilize, the player will continue to be monitored at regular intervals but shall not return to practice, play, or perform any other type of physical activity that day.

Findings of this initial assessment and serial monitoring will be recorded on a *Sideline Head Injury Evaluation Card* (see attachments) or on a similar smart phone application which can later be transferred into the S-A's medical record.

The Emergency Action Plan shall be initiated and the S-A should be removed from the venue utilizing c-spine precautions as needed and transported to the closest emergency department if any of the following are present:

- Prolonged Loss of Consciousness (LOC)
- Focal neurologic defect as found with intracranial injury
- Repeated or worsening emesis
- Significant alteration or deterioration in mental status
- Glasgow Coma Scale score of less than 13

Sub-Acute Evaluation (Controlled/Quiet Environment— Ideally within 1–2 Hours of Injury)

After the initial acute evaluation, the clinician shall perform a more in-depth evaluation of the head injured athlete in a more stable environment such as the Athletic Training Room, locker room or clinic. The *Assessment of Concussion* form shall be utilized for this evaluation (see attachments). This form includes a graded symptom checklist that should be completed by the S-A with assistance of the clinician as needed. Depending on the time elapsed since the SAC was initially administered in the acute evaluation, another SAC may be required. Additional neurological exams will take place to evaluate the status of the S-A. If the clinician is a physician, the form should be completed in its entirety, if the clinician is an athletic trainer, the form shall be completed as fully as possible with the understanding that some of the assessments will not be carried out. If the athlete reports to be symptom free and the remainder of the exam is normal, the clinician may choose to engage the athlete in exertional maneuvers and then reassess symptoms.

Also at this time, a care plan will be discussed. If this sub-acute exam was not completed by a team physician, a follow-up physician exam will be required as soon as possible (and within 48 hours). Depending on signs and symptoms from this sub-acute exam, the clinician may opt to require the S-A to be observed at a health care facility. (On-Campus Health Services, Local Hospital) If the S-A is allowed to return to their room, specific timing and location of the next follow-up exam will be discussed with the S-A. Further, the S-A and another responsible adult will be provided with the *Concussion Home Instruction Sheet* (see attachments) and will be provided with contact information and instructions in the event that the S-A's condition worsens. The clinician should review the home instructions with the S-A, with emphasis given to cautions regarding medication (no NSAIDs) and activity levels, both physical and cognitive (see below).

Sub-Acute Care and "Return-to-Learn"

Along with the follow-up exam already mentioned above, the S-A will be instructed in appropriate behaviors in order to maximize healing conditions for concussion. This will include continued physical rest and also cognitive rest. The athlete will be instructed to limit reading, "screen time" (texting, video game play, computer work) and any other cognitive activity that requires focus/concentration. Learning Resources for Student Athletes (LRSA) will be alerted to the extent of the injury in order to assist with the cognitive rest recommendations. The athlete will be required to discuss a "Return to Learn" plan with both Team Physicians and their LRSA Learning Specialist Advisor who will serve as the "point person" for handling needed academic accommodations. If needed the athlete may initially be housed in a low-sensory environment at University Health Services if cognitive activity increases symptoms. The goal of LRSA and team physicians will be to assist the S-A to minimize cognitive stress while making an attempt to stay current academically. The LRSA Advisor shall make recommendations regarding the resumption of class work and class attendance in a gradual fashion for a period of up to two weeks. In their ongoing monitoring of the concussed S-A, the team physicians, in conjunction with the LRSA Advisor, will make recommendations for continued or increased assistance from University staff as well as off-campus resources to assist with any prolonged Return-to-Learn issues that might continue beyond the initial two week period post-injury. However, increased assistance may be sought out at any time during the monitoring of the S-A's recovery as determined by team physicians or the LRSA Advisor. All recommendations suggested by on-campus and/or off-campus clinicians shall adhere to the ADA Amendments Act of 2008. On-campus resources include Disability Services Office, The Connors Learning Center, University Counseling Services and Office of the Academic Deans. Off-campus resources would initially include the Concussion Neuropsychology Group at Children's Hospital with referral to other expert clinicians as needed.

Follow-Up Evaluation and Care

The concussed S-A shall be re-evaluated within (or close to) 24 hours post injury. At this time, the *Concussion Follow-Up Assessment Form and Self-Report Symptom Scale* document will be utilized for the exam (see attachments). All clinicians should note that on this form the self-report symptom scale is **NOT** graded on **severity of symptoms** but rather on **duration of symptoms**. This must be explained carefully to the S-A and a time frame for symptom report must be selected and noted on the form. Because the scale is different than that employed during the sub-acute exam, the total symptom score should not be compared between these two exams.

When utilizing this follow-up form, the clinician should take into account the timing of the administration of the self-report in regards to the length of time that the S-A has been awake and whether or not the S-A is utilizing any medication that may mitigate symptoms. The form should be completed with care being taken to note any changes in the S-A's condition as well as documentation of the next time and location for serial follow-up evaluation.

Daily monitoring of the concussed S-A shall continue and the *Concussion Follow-Up Assessment Form and Self-Report Symptom Scale* shall again be employed during these evaluations.

ImPACT neurocognitive testing will be carried out on physician recommendation only after the acute and sub-acute symptoms have resolved and the athlete has completed at least the initial two steps of the Return to Play Protocol. The athlete should not undergo ImPACT testing during the initial post-injury phase. Comparison of the ImPACT scores will be made with baseline scores if available or with normative data. The neurocognitive testing results will assist the overall evaluation of the S-A but will not serve as the only measure of progress nor as the only indicator for return to play clearance.

The team physicians shall continue daily monitoring until such as time as the S-A has successfully completed all evaluations, testing values have returned to levels at or near baseline and the S-A has successfully completed the Return-to-Play progression outlined below. If the S-A is experiencing a prolonged recovery and has not been cleared to return to play and/or is still experiencing cognition issues related to Return-To-Learn, team physicians shall convene to discuss additional differential diagnoses as well as other evaluative and care options. As described previously, off-campus resources would initially include the Concussion Neuropsychology Group at Children's Hospital with referral to other expert clinicians as needed.

RETURN TO PLAY CONSIDERATIONS

The Return to Play (RTP) protocol following a concussion follows a step-wise progression and is not initiated until approximately 24 hours after the S-A is asymptomatic and other neurological evaluations are considered back to normal. A physician must approve the commencement of the RTP progression. The progression outlined below is to be carried out in a step-wise fashion with constant monitoring both before and after activity by a sports medicine clinician. The *Concussion Follow-Up Assessment Form and Self-Report Symptom Scale* will be used again after each step. If recurrence of symptoms is noted and/or a change in the neurological exam occurs, the athlete will again be held from activity for approximately 24 hours and re-evaluated. If the symptoms have resolved, the athlete will drop back to the previous step and be allowed to resume the progression. Integration of two steps within a 24 hour period is permissible only with physician approval.

Step 1—Light aerobic exercise to increase heart rate (walking, stationary bike, elliptical, etc.)
Step 2—Sport specific cardio activity (ex: skating, running)
Step 3—Progressive resistance exercise
Step 4—Non-contact practice
Step 5—Return to full contact play with clearance by physician

*While self-evident when following all of the guidelines outlined in this document, it should be noted that at no time will a S-A be allowed to return to play if they still require academic adaptations or accommodations related to their concussion.

Special Considerations

The sports medicine clinician may consider obtaining a neurological consult or an adjustment of the RTP progression in certain situations. Find below a list of some of those situations that may warrant a change in the normal protocol.

Structural Head Injury

• Multiple Concussions
• Extensive duration of symptoms at any point post injury
• Significant amnesia or LOC greater than 1 minute
• Comorbidities such as a past history medical history of migraine, depression, ADHD, sleep disorder, and/or other mental health issues

Summary

It is important to note that concussion evaluation and management must be handled on a case-by- case basis. There is no "typical" clinical course for the resolution of the injury itself and the post concussive management. In following the mission of Boston College Sports Medicine, we will protect and promote the safety, health, and well-being of every student athlete and will provide and coordinate the care of our athletes while working with our coaches as they prepare for athletic competition. Post concussive care will focus on limiting the potential catastrophic and long term risks involved with concussive injuries. The evaluation, care and return to play decisions will be based on current best medical practices and the clinical judgments made by Boston College clinicians specifically for each injured individual.

The above policy and protocols will be reviewed by the Director of Health Services, the Medical Director of Athletics, Team Physicians and Sports Medicine Staff. This review will occur yearly in July and the policy will be updated to reflect current best-practices for care of head-injured athletes. Further, the policy and protocol will be reviewed and updated at any time as needed to insure that the document meets the requirements of all governing bodies including but not limited to; the University, the National Collegiate Athletic Association, the City of Boston, and the City of Newton.

EMERGENCY ACTION PLANS

Find following the Emergency Action Plans (EAPs) for the various venues utilized by Boston College athletic teams for both practices and competitions.

It should be noted the Emergency Action Plans are venue (site) specific. They are **not** sport specific, nor are they activity specific (i.e., practice v. game v. running workout v. coaches skill work, etc.), nor are they injury specific (i.e., concussion v. cardiac v. orthopedic, etc.)

The EAPs are documents to be used by any individuals or groups affiliated with Boston College that are using a Boston College athletic venue, or an off-campus public or private venue utilized by Boston College athletic teams. The plans are designed to assist on-site staff in the event of any type of medical emergency. The EAP is specifically designed to be direct, succinct and related only to initial emergent care. *The EAP is not a protocol for dealing with specific injuries or conditions.* (See related documents for policies and protocols regarding specific injuries or conditions.)

All staff utilizing venues should be familiar with the EAP for that venue. When possible, the EAP will be posted in a prominent location at each venue.

Emergency Action Plans Attached:

Alumni Stadium
Community Rowing Boat House
Conte Forum: Main Floor or Ice Surface
Conte Forum: Power Gymnasium
Flynn Recreational Complex
Newton Campus Short Turf Field
Newton Campus Long Turf Field
Savin Hill Yacht Club
Shea Field

Boston College Sports Medicine

Concussion Assessment Form

Name _____ Sport _____ Eagle ID _____

Date of Injury _____ Time of Injury _____

Date of Exam _____ Time of Exam _____

Mechanism of Injury (briefly)_____

Does patient have a history of prior concussions: No or Yes, When _____

Current Symptoms	None	Mild		Moderate		Severe	
Headache	0	1	2	3	4	5	6
Nausea	0	1	2	3	4	5	6
Balance difficulty/dizziness	0	1	2	3	4	5	6
Fatigue	0	1	2	3	4	5	6
Drowsiness	0	1	2	3	4	5	6
Feeling like "in a fog"	0	1	2	3	4	5	6
Difficulty concentrating	0	1	2	3	4	5	6
Difficulty remembering	0	1	2	3	4	5	6
Sensitivity to light	0	1	2	3	4	5	6
Sensitivity to noise	0	1	2	3	4	5	6
Visual Changes (blurry, spots, etc.)	0	1	2	3	4	5	6
Feeling "slowed down"	0	1	2	3	4	5	6

Total Symptom Score _____

Loss of Consciousness: No or Yes, Duration _____

Amnesia: Pre Injury No or Yes, Duration _____

Amnesia: Post Injury No or Yes, Duration _____

BP _____ Pulse _____ Glasgow Score _____ Tympanic Membrane Clear: No or Yes

Neurological Exam

Pupils equal: No or Yes   Pupils reactive: No or Yes

Fundi: Normal or Abnormal, Finding: _____

Central Nerves II–VII Normal or Abnormal, Finding: _____

    Motor   Normal or Abnormal, Finding: _____

    Sensory   Normal or Abnormal, Finding: _____

    Deep Tendon Reflex Normal or Abnormal, Finding _____

Balance Score: Eyes Open 10 sec. Stance Rt. Leg: No or Yes, Lt. Leg: No or Yes

(Perform Barefoot) Eyes Closed 10 sec. Stance Rt. Leg: No or Yes, Lt. Leg: No or Yes

Tandem Gait, 5 ft: No or Yes

SAC Score _____ Baseline SAC Score _____

Comments/Plan: _____

_____

_____

_____ Clinician _____

Follow-up On: _____ Location: _____

Boston College Sports Medicine

Concussion Follow-Up Assessment and Self Report Symptom Scale

Name _____ Eagle ID _____

Today's Date ____ Date of Injury _____ Current Time of Day_____ AM/PM

Please complete the following scale based on how you have felt for the past_____days/hours and/or Now

Symptom	Never		Sometimes				Always		NOW	
Headache	0	1	2	3	4	5	6		Yes	No
Nausea	0	1	2	3	4	5	6		Yes	No
Balance difficulty/dizziness	0	1	2	3	4	5	6		Yes	No
Fatigue	0	1	2	3	4	5	6		Yes	No
Drowsiness	0	1	2	3	4	5	6		Yes	No
Feeling like "in a fog"	0	1	2	3	4	5	6		Yes	No
Difficulty concentrating	0	1	2	3	4	5	6		Yes	No
Difficulty remembering	0	1	2	3	4	5	6		Yes	No
Sensitivity to light	0	1	2	3	4	5	6		Yes	No
Sensitivity to noise	0	1	2	3	4	5	6		Yes	No
Visual Changes (blurry, spots, etc.)	0	1	2	3	4	5	6		Yes	No
Feeling "slowed down"	0	1	2	3	4	5	6		Yes	No

Sleeping more than normal last night or today if you took a nap?   No or Yes

Did you have trouble falling asleep, or staying asleep last night, or today if you tried to take a nap? No or Yes

Balance Score: **Eyes Open 10 sec. Stance** *Rt. Leg*: No or Yes, *Lt. Leg*: No or Yes
(Perform Barefoot)
> **Eyes Closed 10 sec. Stance** *Rt. Leg*: No or Yes, *Lt. Leg*: No or Yes
> **Tandem Gait, 5 ft.**: No or Yes

Impact Test Needed (only at end of progression): No or Yes, Date/Time:____

Today's Neurological Exam and/or Comments: _____
_____
_____
_____
_____

Plan: _____
_____

_____ Examining Clinician: _____

Follow-up: When _____ Where _____ With _____

BOSTON COLLEGE SPORTS MEDICINE

CONCUSSION HOME INSTRUCTION SHEET

Name: _____ Date: _____

Please follow the recommendations below to ensure a safe recovery from your injury.

Please report to: _____ for your next follow-up appointment with _____ which will take place on _____ at _____ o'clock.

If any of the following symptoms get worse before the above appointment time, please report to Health Services in Cushing Hall or call Boston College Campus Police at 617-552-4444.

- Decreasing level of consciousness
- Increasing severity of headache
- Confusion or change of mental status
- Seizure
- Vomiting

It's OK to:	There's no need to:	DO NOT:
- Use acetaminophen (Tylenol) for headaches	- Check eyes with a flashlight	- Drink alcohol
	- Test reflexes	- Take aspirin or ibuprofen
- Use ice pack on head and neck for comfort	- Stay in bed	- Read/text/play video games
- Go to sleep / rest		- Engage in strenuous activity

SERIES AFTERWORD

Over the past 100 years, there have been incredible medical breakthroughs that have prevented or cured illness in billions of people and helped many more improve their health while living with chronic conditions. A few of the most important 20th-century discoveries include antibiotics, organ transplants, and vaccines. The 21st century has already heralded important new treatments including a vaccine to prevent human papillomavirus from infecting and potentially leading to cervical cancer in women. Polio is on the verge of being eradicated worldwide, making it only the second infectious disease behind smallpox to ever be erased as a human health threat.

In this series, experts from many disciplines share with readers important information about medical issues—including problems, symptoms, diseases, and whenever possible, solutions. Disseminating this information will help individuals to recognize things that impact their health and that of loved ones. Researchers may use these books to determine where there are gaps in our current knowledge, and policy makers may be able to better assess the most pressing needs in health care. The overarching goal of this series of books is to inform people about important issues in modern medicine.

Series Editor Julie K. Silver, MD
Associate Professor and Associate Chair
Department of Physical Medicine and Rehabilitation
Harvard Medical School

INDEX

About the Author

WILLIAM PAUL MEEHAN III, MD, is director of the Micheli Center for Sports Injury Prevention and director of Research for the Brain Injury Center at Boston Children's Hospital. He graduated from Harvard Medical School, where he is currently an associate professor of pediatrics and orthopedics. He conducts both clinical and scientific research in the area of sports injuries and concussive brain injury. His research has been funded by the National Institutes of Health, the Center for the Integration of Medicine and Innovative Technology, the National Football League Players Association, the National Football League, and the National Hockey League Alumni Association. He is the 2012 winner of the American Medical Society for Sports Medicine's award for Best Overall Research. He has more than 100 medical and scientific publications, is co-editor of the book *Head and Neck Injuries in Young Athletes*, and is author of the books *Kids, Sports, and Concussion: A Guide for Coaches and Parents*, first edition, and *Concussions*.